D0710827

Praise for *The Socially Included Child*

"This book has practical solutions and great strategies that will no doubt help you and your kids get out and enjoy!"

—Jenny McCarthy, *New York Times* bestselling author

"This book is an indispensable resource to empower parents with practical, hands-on help as we seek to reconnect our kids with the real world."   —Lynn M. Hamilton, parent and author of *Facing Autism: Giving Parents Reasons for Hope and Guidance for Help*

"Chock-full of practical methods for teaching children with autism. Great for both parents and teachers."

—Temple Grandin, author of *Thinking in Pictures*

"When you're the parent of a child with autism, you know how vitally important it is to increase your child's social skills—and how challenging a task that can be. Thankfully, LeComer offers concrete strategies for facilitating your child's social interactions."

—Claire LaZebnik, coauthor of *Overcoming Autism* and *Growing Up on the Spectrum*

"Children with autism and autism spectrum disorders can benefit significantly from inclusion in family, community, and school activities . . . Parents and family members will find this an invaluable resource."   —Fred R. Volkmar, M.D., Director, Yale Child Study Center

"LeComer truly 'gets it,' as my son would say, and has come up with practical, easy-to-use strategies to make social activities successful for the child with autism and enjoyable for everyone else. Knowing your child and planning for these events is key. The I.D.E.A.L system LeComer has developed is a great tool. I highly recommend this book."   —Chantal Sicile-Kira, author of *Autism Life Skills*

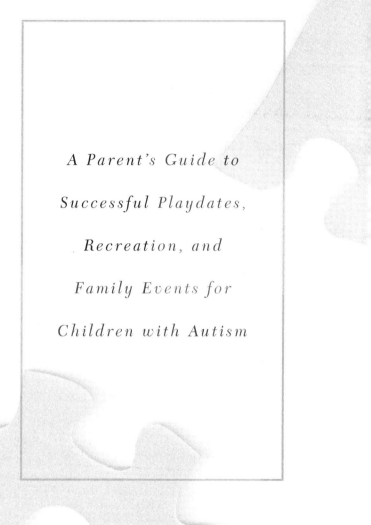

A Parent's Guide to

Successful Playdates,

Recreation, and

Family Events for

Children with Autism

Most Berkley Books are available at special quantity discounts for bulk purchases for sales promotions, premiums, fund-raising, or educational use. Special books, or book excerpts, can also be created to fit specific needs.
For details, write: Special Markets, The Berkley Publishing Group, 375 Hudson Street, New York, New York 10014.

The Socially Included Child

Laurie LeComer, M.Ed.

BERKLEY BOOKS,
NEW YORK

THE BERKLEY PUBLISHING GROUP
Published by the Penguin Group
Penguin Group (USA) Inc.
375 Hudson Street, New York, New York 10014, USA
Penguin Group (Canada), 90 Eglinton Avenue East, Suite 700, Toronto, Ontario M4P 2Y3, Canada
(a division of Pearson Penguin Canada Inc.)
Penguin Books Ltd., 80 Strand, London WC2R 0RL, England
Penguin Group Ireland, 25 St. Stephen's Green, Dublin 2, Ireland (a division of Penguin Books Ltd.)
Penguin Group (Australia), 250 Camberwell Road, Camberwell, Victoria 3124, Australia
(a division of Pearson Australia Group Pty. Ltd.)
Penguin Books India Pvt. Ltd., 11 Community Centre, Panchsheel Park, New Delhi—110 017, India
Penguin Group (NZ), 67 Apollo Drive, Rosedale, North Shore 0632, New Zealand
(a division of Pearson New Zealand Ltd.)
Penguin Books (South Africa) (Pty.) Ltd., 24 Sturdee Avenue, Rosebank, Johannesburg 2196, South Africa

Penguin Books Ltd., Registered Offices: 80 Strand, London WC2R 0RL, England

This book is an original publication of The Berkley Publishing Group.

PUBLISHER'S NOTE: Every effort has been made to ensure that the information contained in this book is complete and accurate. However, neither the publisher nor the author is engaged in rendering professional advice or services to the individual reader. The ideas, procedures, and suggestions contained in this book are not intended as a substitute for consulting with your physician. All matters regarding your health require medical supervision. Neither the author nor the publisher shall be liable or responsible for any loss or damage allegedly arising from any information or suggestion in this book.

The events described in this book are the real experiences of real people. However, the author has altered their identities and, in some instances, created composite characters. Any resemblance between a character in this book and a real person therefore is entirely accidental.

While the author has made every effort to provide accurate telephone numbers and Internet addresses at the time of publication, neither the publisher nor the author assumes any responsibility for errors, or for changes that occur after publication. Further, the publisher does not have any control over and does not assume any responsibility for author or third-party websites or their content.

Copyright © 2009 by Laurie LeComer.
Cover design by Pyrographx.
Cover photograph by Shutterstock.
Text design by Ellen Cipriano.

All rights reserved.
No part of this book may be reproduced, scanned, or distributed in any printed or electronic form without permission. Please do not participate in or encourage piracy of copyrighted materials in violation of the author's rights. Purchase only authorized editions.
BERKLEY® is a registered trademark of Penguin Group (USA) Inc.
The "B" design is a trademark of Penguin Group (USA) Inc.

PRINTING HISTORY
Berkley trade paperback edition / December 2009

Library of Congress Cataloging-in-Publication Data

LeComer, Laurie.
    The socially included child / Laurie LeComer.
       p.   cm.
    ISBN 978-0-425-22965-1
    1. Autistic children.   2. Socialization.   I. Title.
    RJ506.A9L435 2009
    618.92'85882—dc22
                                    2009019181

PRINTED IN THE UNITED STATES OF AMERICA

10   9   8   7   6   5   4   3   2   1

For my sister, Karen, and my nephew and hero, Ben

And for Gavi, Darnell, Dana, Sarah, Tony, Ethan, and Dylan, who unknowingly, but brilliantly, inspired this book

ACKNOWLEDGMENTS

There are many people who put their special touches into the pages of this book. My inspiration for this work came from some wonderful kids with autism—I wish all of you could have the pleasure of meeting them. They struggle daily, but are role models to all they come across, through their joy, humor, and strength. Each child has taught me unique and important lessons, and I thank them for those lessons and their company and love.

I am very thankful for the guidance of my agent, Judith Riven, and am greatly appreciative of her work on my behalf. And I am also grateful this book landed in the hands of my editor, Adrienne Avila, whose sound suggestions, deep interest, and intuitive understanding of the subject made this a better book. Thanks also to my publisher, Leslie Gelbman, and the staff at Berkley Books.

I am extremely grateful to those who had to live with me during the book writing process—my helpful and supportive husband, Victor, and my kids, Ian, Tyler, and Paige. And thanks to my father, Sherman Fivozinsky, and his wife (my friend) Carol Fivozinsky, for their support and uplifting conversations.

To Stephanie Vullo and Paula Schwartz, thanks so much for

your friendship—I hope we can continue to watch our kids work their magic together. And thanks to Fred Volkmar, M.D., Jenny McCarthy, Temple Grandin, Claire LaZebnik, Chantal Sicile-Kira, and Lynn Hamilton, for their support of this project. I appreciate so very much the time (and vacation time!) spent on this book's behalf.

Many other friends and colleagues have challenged and inspired me: Leslie Bernstein, Melissa O'Connell, Lucia Green, Douglas Rushkoff, Rachel Fleishman, Lisa Horowitz, Melinda Gardiner, Ellen Talley Lotsky, Julie Seen, Joan Villegas, Joann White, Kristen Mosher, Carole MacDonald, Meg Barlow, Douglas Martung, Connie Mandrozos, Mike Abraham, Jacalyn Papstein, Stephanie Miklos, Lisa Norcross, Ann-Marie Soto, Sarah Stevens, Carol Bloch, Marybeth Buckwald, Liz Horvath, Liz Finck, Alyson Martin, Beth Lukas, Catherine Rotundi, Cathy Lambert, Jessica Woods, and Kathy Smith.

Also, a gracious, heartfelt thank-you to Carol Sissala, Easter Seals Treatment Center of Montgomery County, Maryland, the staff at Georgetown University Hospital, and Scarsdale public schools.

Thanks so much to my sister, Karen Feibus, for our discussions—and the intelligent suggestions that helped keep me sane through many long nights. And thanks to Jon Feibus for the much-needed brotherly support.

Lastly, I would like to give a special thank-you to the parents I have come to know well, and who were gracious enough to share their stories.

CONTENTS

PART TWO

Previewing and Planning Using I.D.E.A.L. Elements

PART THREE

Facilitating Social Opportunities Using I.D.E.A.L.

Introduction

Today, a young student of mine with autism—Jeremy—approached a typical peer with the intention of initiating a social interaction. Jeremy has little language, and is unable to comfortably use his functional language with peers, but he donned a favorite cat puppet on his hand and approached another boy in the student support center. I, along with the other adults in the room, froze with bated anticipation—and hope—for a successful initiation and a positive outcome for him. Jeremy's efforts were new and exciting, but he had the comfort of embarking on this challenge in the relaxed atmosphere of his familiar, everyday environment. Jeremy was among people he had come to know well.

With little skips he approached the peer and grinned. He then took his cat puppet and gently opened and closed its mouth against the peer's shoulder, as if the cat were nibbling the peer's shoulder. The peer immediately smiled and exclaimed out loud with glee, "Jeremy's making the cat eat my arm! Did you see that?" Jeremy repeated the munching action (now excited) with a munching sound, and both boys laughed together. To the naked eye, this may not seem like a great feat, but to those of us who have worked long and hard with Jeremy, it was better than Christmas. Jeremy did it. He took the initiative and moved past his communicative deficits and sensory processing difficulties for a beautiful moment of shared joy and friendship.

I began working with children with autism in 1983 at an Easter Seals Treatment Center outside Washington, D.C. The children I worked with were nonverbal, and were incorporated into special needs classes of ten to twelve kids with multiple types of disabilities. At the time, autism seemed to be a rare and mysterious childhood affliction that robbed children of the desire to interact in "our" world. I remember joining one severely affected little boy's play of tapping objects in the room with plastic belts. I would follow him and tap what he tapped. We did this together for long periods of time, and then I had the idea to tap his shoes, and he followed suit and tapped mine. This was the beginning of our communication—our ability to begin to request and respond to one another, but our bond had formed long before anyone would be able to officially take note. Even with the autistic little ones way back then, I was aware of the kids' desire to connect in some way—albeit their own way— with others. Even then, I didn't believe that children with autism choose to live solitary lives. And I don't believe it now. Like all of us, children with autism move toward what feels most comfortable to them.

Over the years, the children I have worked with have been in both public and private settings. I often received children right after their diagnosis. I was someone the children were sent to—to begin their learning, their progress, or their recovery (depending on how the pediatrician presented their prognosis). It was up to me to make things happen. Make the children less autistic, so to speak. Over time, a frustration started growing in me, as children with autism would come to me with psychological, functional, and academic evaluations that did not and could not tell the story of who they really were. They would arrive with recommendations for improved communication ability, improved social understanding, and more advanced skills in activities of daily living—with no suggestions on how to help each individual child move forward. One autistic kindergartener came to me with the general recommendation to replace behaviors that were interfering with his learning—I had to initially retreat to a bathroom to work with this little boy, for he would tantrum when the classroom lights were turned on. He was also one of the sweetest, brightest little guys you could meet. I was left to search and experiment. Many professional colleagues were willing to discuss what *should* be done with kids, but few were willing to discuss the specifics of *how* to get children from point A to point B, from dysfunction to function.

"Behavioral modification techniques should be used" was commonly voiced, or written on menu-like lists of general and impersonal suggestions. And as the number of children with autism on my caseload grew, so did my fascination with the many different ways kids were affected by the disorder. I joined professional organizations, recruited for national studies, and became a member of the Harvard Graduate School of Education's Collaborative on Integrated School Services, which inspired ideas used in my program for children with autism, OASIS (Optimal Academic and Social Instructional Sessions), where children with autism are integrated with typical peers into small settings for shorter academic and social "sessions."

However, there was no one answer, no "one size fits all" strategy. What worked for one did not work for another. And what worked for another did not work for the next. The need to individualize the approach to socialization for each child was apparent, and it was through this learning, from preparing for and implementing social instructional sessions for many different children with autism, that the I.D.E.A.L. system for social inclusion was born.

The value of I.D.E.A.L. is felt in its practicality and in its ability to be individualized for any child on the spectrum. I.D.E.A.L. can be used for any autistic person who has not reached social independence or who struggles with sensory, communicative, or self-regulatory issues, although this book is geared more toward the young child or youth with autism (two to eleven years old)—for that is where my experience lies. It has been exciting to see what a difference a simple preparation and organizational tool can make at school, at home, and in the community. I.D.E.A.L. has helped children who have not typically been able to join in with others to finally begin to participate in social activities and events. I.D.E.A.L. has helped children with higher-functioning autism to feel more at ease in social situations through better preparation, self-regulation, and increased independence.

Children and adults with autism are now members of all our communities. But I was still shocked by the Center for Disease Control's 2007 announcement that autism now affects 1 in every 150 kids. It is truly hard to believe how many of us are now touched by the disorder in our families, communities, work, or close friendships. On a daily basis, I find myself in discussions with others who care deeply about the well-being of loved ones afflicted with autism spectrum disorders (ASDs), and within these conversations, there seems to be a shared anxiety rooted in our frantic search for answers we are currently unable to find. Autism still holds that mystery. Even with the recent attention on autism, interventions, and the progress made in determining some possible causes, there continues to be so much—too much—that remains unknown.

Socialization

Socialization has become an issue of extreme importance for families of children with autism. Many parents worry and fear for their children's futures as they observe the multiple types of struggles their children endure in social situations. We know how much social skills come into play both in our personal and work lives, but the difficulties and stress parents of children with autism experience when they try to pull off something as simple as a playdate for their child can often rival the preparation involved in the planning of a wedding. Isn't it true that at a wedding rehearsal the hope is that, despite everyone's frayed nerves, anxious moods, and high expectations, the practice will ultimately help the event run smoothly, with a minimum of slip-ups? This heightened stress and trepidation are what many parents of children with autism *routinely* feel when readying themselves and their children to participate in everyday social events and activities.

For children with autism, birthday parties and noisy family events can become hectic and painful, and some parents find the preparation and/or embarrassment too hard to endure, so they repeatedly pass up opportunities to connect.

The struggle to find ways to socially include their children with autism has brought many parents to tears, and this is why we need to look further, try harder, and devise better methods to make this socialization happen more easily and systematically.

Studies have shown that it is important for autistic children to navigate natural social environments to learn social skills and tolerance skills. But parents continually find themselves faced with the dilemmas of:

- Finding peers their children can play with (which involves finding parents who are willing to allow their children to act as ambassadors)

- Finding safe activities their children can take part in

- Finding ways to exert some control in overwhelming or overstimulating environments

- Finding peers in their child's age group who have similar interests to those of their child

Assisting Our Children in Natural Social Environments

It is very common for children who learn in quiet, structured environments and discrete trial settings to find generalizing skills problematic, especially when social in nature. Though a child may be able to, for example, learn appropriate social phrases, learn to share, and practice better eye contact with a teacher or an ABA provider, the generalization of skills such as these can be difficult.

This is why it is so important for children with autism to gain some familiarity with the sounds and aesthetic feels of social activities. With exposure over time, even when involvement is limited, children will gain a degree of comfort and familiarity with different settings and expectations, which can bring about further participation and desensitization to new sensory experiences.

For children with extremely difficult behaviors, simply eating a snack among others, or retrieving a favorite book or toy in the midst of others in a natural setting, can begin the journey of increased social comfort. Even brief bits of exposure, one experience at a time, to natural social environments can plant the seeds for the growth of increased comfort, enjoyment, and participation among others.

This book will help you learn to prepare and plan for these social moments, including playdates, family outings, and more.

The Challenges Kids and Parents Face

For children with autism, just the sights and sounds of people interacting can be overwhelming. Robbie and Luke are two six-year-old boys with autism, who struggle daily to interact with adults and peers:

- Robbie has very little eye contact and is often withdrawn, but he shows interest in others through inappropriate actions such as poking and hitting. At parties, Robbie will grab at food and wrapped presents, and will tantrum if someone tries to remove food or toys from his hands. When Robbie acts out inappropriately toward other peers, his parents become extremely anxious and apologetic. Consequently, they avoid most parties and family get-togethers. They believe Robbie is not yet ready to handle being among a group.

- Luke also has very little eye contact, but does use some simple language to express wants and needs. Luke is very small and physically beautiful, so he tends to attract more peer interest, and has received some invites to birthday parties from classmates. If there is a lot of noise or commotion at parties, however, Luke, who has extreme sensitivities to sound, will "melt down" (screaming, kicking, and hyperventilating). His parents have turned down most of the invitations because of the stress involved in bringing him. Luke is also on a special casein-free diet, which has made eating away from home very difficult. Luke's parents worry about how their avoidance of social outings and entertaining will affect Luke's developmentally normal twin sister, Brittany.

• Andrew also struggles in social situations. Andrew is seven years old, and has autism that is considered to be moderate to severe. He recently had several harrowing experiences with family members in public places that had emotionally lasting effects on his mom and a potential friend. The first difficult situation occurred on a family beach trip. Upon arrival at the beach, Andrew bolted from the family's parked car and ran across the sand toward the water. He lost his balance at the shoreline and fell into the waves. He did not know how to swim. Luckily, an alert beachgoer moved quickly to get Andrew out of the water. The horror of this potentially life-threatening experience still haunts Andrew's mother to this day. It has made her reluctant to include Andrew on family outings. A second incident happened recently when Andrew's mom brought Andrew and a peer to the mall so that they could go to a Build-a-Bear store. At the entrance, Andrew refused to go in, and when Andrew's mother tried to talk with him, and get him to follow the "friend" into the store, Andrew became agitated and punched at a stranger (a woman) standing close by. Then he bolted. Andrew's mother had Andrew's little sister and the young peer with her, and had to run off after Andrew in the mall to catch him.

It is situations like these that cause parents to think twice about bringing their children with autism out into public domains—outside of their children's homes and school programs; outside of their structured activities and routines.

Why This Book

Parents of children who exhibit difficult behaviors or extreme sensitivities, such as Robbie, Luke, and Andrew, want to help their children navigate the social world of interacting with friends, family, and the general public. Yet all too often, the child's needs or behaviors end up isolating the *entire* family. The current information available for parents on socially including their kids with autism is very education oriented, offering one-on-one lessons in language and play development. These skills, in many cases, take months or even years to develop, and this realization leaves many parents feeling hopeless. Sadly, many parents are left with a sense that their children cannot be included until they display appropriate language and play skills.

I want you to know that your child will not have to perform at certain language, play, or reciprocity skill levels to benefit from the information in this book. He will be able to begin to participate socially from whatever level he is currently at, and with whatever behaviors he brings to a situation. You will be able to move forward from right where you are.

One parent I know believed that her autistic son responded only to RDI (Relationship Development Intervention) techniques of relating. This belief made her want all teachers, therapists, school personnel, and children in his school to be "trained" in this very specific technique. As you can imagine, it is not realistic to "train" all who come into contact with an autistic child.

But it is possible to prepare, and it is my hope that this book will help guide you as you work to give positive social experiences to your children with autism. This book will show you how to quickly address the elements needed, to plan and carry out successful social activities in natural settings. The I.D.E.A.L. system will allow you to individualize your preparations and approaches to accommodate your own child's unique characteristics, tolerance levels, and skills, so that she can participate in positive social experiences that she can build upon.

And in *The Socially Included Child*, I will not just tell you to include your child more; I will show you how. I will not just tell you to use behavior modification techniques to decrease behaviors; I will explain some options and how they may work for your child. If you are one of the many parents who have experienced feelings of isolation, I hope this book will empower you to reenter the "real world" with your child.

How to Use This Book

This is not a book that will give you a general introduction to autism and its symptoms—though symptoms and how they affect socialization will be discussed. Nor will I describe what each autism spectrum disorder looks like. This is a book that will give you a wealth of information and strategies through clear action steps that will help to foster better social experiences within natural social environments for your child, and possibly the whole family.

In my work, I have focused on some key, universal issues in preparing and accommodating kids with autism for social activities that can be addressed in a systematic approach no matter the child's level of severity. This approach consists of five simple but powerful action steps that together make up the system of I.D.E.A.L.

Part One of this book will guide you through the many different expectations and issues that affect social success. Anecdotes will be included, along with clear explanations and individualized exercises. I will guide you as we look at your child's stamina, sensory processing, modes of communication, interests, and approachability.

Part Two will introduce the exciting new tool, the I.D.E.A.L. system, which will help you preview, plan, and carry out social activities. By using this new organizational tool, you will learn to:

- **I**ntroduce an activity.

- **D**etermine the tasks involved.

- **E**valuate your expectations.

- **A**ccommodate for success.

- **L**ist the activity components visually.

Part Three will address in detail how to facilitate specific social events (using I.D.E.A.L.) such as birthday parties, playdates, and family events.

You Are Not Alone

A few years ago, I sat knee-to-knee with an autistic five-year-old student of mine—a very bright but echolalic and challenging boy. We were impressed with his ability to learn academic skills, but had great concern and frustration with his lack of interest in peers and low sensory tolerance. I had just been teaching him some social phrases using social scripts and visuals, when I was suddenly overwhelmed with the thought of how hard it must be for him to constantly be put into uncomfortable situations (groups of people/noisy environments) while being prompted (prodded?) to participate and attend. This child's individualized educational plan (IEP) was loaded with social objectives that would consistently expect more than this child was able to tolerate or perform. If he mastered his social objectives, however, he would indeed appear quite typical.

I remember thinking that the adult expectations were an element that would need to be addressed as part of a successful plan to move children forward from where they truly were—and how unbelievably easier it is to write an objective on paper than to work day by day on increasing sensory tolerance and decreasing self-stimulation behaviors. The little guy sitting in front of me (who bonked me on the leg, wondering why I had stopped saying my portion of the script) would need to start small—incrementally small—and move forward from there.

Of course we should have high expectations for our kids—we should for all kids—but it is important to break up larger lessons and more challenging situations into more doable chunks, which are the right sizes and amounts for each individual child to handle. Every child should be able to feel a little degree of success each and every day.

This is the real thing. As part of the I.D.E.A.L. process, you will be taking a closer, more in-depth look at your own child. For those of you involved in the maze of diagnosis information, IEP advice, and modified educational curriculums, I know that the issues of *quality of life, friendship, independence*, and *the ability to deal in "the real world"* are at the forefront of your thoughts for your child. And you are not alone. Throughout the special needs community, the need and the desire for helpful information in this regard are very strong.

It is my hope that the importance and value of *The Socially Included Child* will resonate with you, whether you are a parent, teacher, therapist, family member, or friend of a child with autism. We truly need to be an extended community working together to make things better for our kids. Few know how difficult it can be, to be on the front lines with our children with autism—in the position of doing the daily work needed, little by little, situation by situation, and negotiating the daily dilemmas that come up.

If you are struggling, and looking for helpful tools that will make your life easier but at the same time will not compromise the extraordinary efforts you make with your child each day, this book is for you.

The foundation skills your child will gain through social activities and experiences will no doubt help her as she grows throughout youth and into young adulthood. As an individual, each child will strive and struggle in her own unique ways. And we will need to help her. In the following pages, I will show you *how*.

Social

Considerations

and Individualized

Expectations

CHAPTER 1

❖ ❖ ❖

Your Child's Interests, Approachability, and Communication Style

When they first moved here, I was afraid of him and I didn't want to go near him. But I know him now, and he can't help it—he's not trying to scare people or not be nice. I play with him sometimes now. I tried to teach him to kick a ball yesterday.

—*KEVIN*, *age nine,*
friend and neighbor of Bryan, who has autism

Typical children who find and maintain friendships have the innate gift of understanding social concepts. They are able to pick up social cues and apply social rules, such as rules of proximity, voice volume, and eye contact. We see children apply these concepts as they initiate conversations, share toys, and take turns during games on the playground. In typical friendships, children enjoy each other's company and share similar interests and communication styles. They even have similar styles of dress.

Children with autism often do not possess this gift. They may not understand social concepts, or know how to initiate and maintain conversations. They may or may not share interests with same-age peers. Most children with autism call negative attention to themselves because their interests and preferred activities—activities they most like to do—look odd or seem like fixations. Sometimes children with autism demand that a game be played one specific way every time, or that a peer or adult take on a same role over and over again.

Typical children do not see this control as fun, and will frequently avoid or stop participating in such rigid play. Typical children have what we call "flexibility," and can gracefully move from one activity to the next while maintaining an appropriate mood and conversation. Children that exhibit flexibility can cooperate even when they don't get their way, and can negotiate their social roles when among others. Flexibility allows for a child to sometimes be the leader and sometimes be the follower.

Why is it so hard for our children with autism to approach peers, join in, and stay for a while? Children with autism have very real differences in their processing and perception, which affect the ways they are experiencing their environments—and all that is going on around them. The puzzling actions and reactions of children with autism can be very disconcerting to both parents and peers. But if we remember that the children are not experiencing activities or locations as we are, we can learn more about and understand what's happening a bit better, and then prepare our children more wisely for new experiences.

As we begin to help our children with autism become more successful in social environments, it is fascinating to look at the many different ways we define social success. Our opinions on social success and what it entails are as individual as our children with autism. Social success for some may mean a lot of friends, and ease among peers—maybe even popularity. Social success for others may mean understanding manners, and when to use them. Some may say the ability to play team sports and display sportsmanship exemplifies social success.

For parents of children with autism, conversations pertaining to social success usually contain phrases such as: showing an awareness of peers; making eye contact with peers; referencing peers; and functioning appropriately in social environments. It is the wish of many parents that their children will be accepted by peers, and that their children will form true friendships—as opposed to simply participating in minimally interactive "role model pairings."

It is my experience that true friendships really can happen for children with autism. Kids with even severe autism can, over time, get to know and feel comfortable with another child—typical or disabled. Friendships take time to form, though, and the growth of *familiarity* in a safe environment is important for children who find typical modes of socialization difficult.

Socializing is truly an amorphous concept as well as an uncomfortable endeavor for most children with autism. And although a common symptom of austim is "showing no interest in peers," most of the children I have worked with over the years clearly did show an interest in the others in their environments. Sometimes young children with autism would show their interest by noticing or tracking others—noticing a peer had picked up a certain preferred object, or had a preferred food; or by tracking where another child was taking a preferred toy. My little friend Kate appropriately sat down at a table to have her snack, while her classmate Michael flopped to the floor in protest. Michael was trying to pull us to the snack food he preferred (graham crackers), but Michael had been prompted to use his words. So, we offered Kate some of the graham crackers, and once Michael noticed, he magically rose and walked to Kate's side and watched her intently as she ate her graham cracker. We then prompted Michael *to ask Kate* for a graham cracker—and he did, using his words. Even though this is an "object-oriented" interest, his attention to and awareness of his peer were clear.

Children with autism often become used to the presence of certain peers in familiar daily activities, and will begin to look for these peers. Many children with autism will begin to speak directly to or gesture directly to familiar peers. Children also learn to use their peers as vehicles to help them get what they want—in the same way they might use a family member to "get" or "reach" for them.

I have seen children with autism form meaningful attachments to family members, teachers, and peers. Some of the interactions may look a little different, but the connectedness is present.

It is my belief that the "want" to be social is there. It is just hard for the kids to understand "the rules of appropriateness" and to overcome the many discomforts and sensitivities they are bombarded with on a daily basis. It isn't easy to remember social scripts, rules, social language, or motor plans when clothing itches, volume levels hurt, or primary needs are not being met due to an inability to communicate. As with all of us, it can be very natural to try to move away from what feels uncomfortable and risky, and move toward what feels comfortable, familiar, and safe.

You may notice me using the word "familiar" often. This is because familiarity is an important "feeling" for children with autism. Growth of social skills can be linked with becoming familiar with certain adults, peers, rules, phrases, and routines. In a familiar environment or with a familiar person, children with autism are more communicatively available for social interaction. It takes time to establish familiarity, so in new social situations and environments, it is important to include familiar persons, objects, or routines. For successful moments of participation to take place, familiar and practiced elements need to be present.

Preferred Activities

Like typical children, children with autism have their own distinct and individual interests. Participation in activities of interest can go hand in hand with feelings of comfort and safety. Though some of these interests may look inappropriate, there are actions and/or activities as well as video or book characters your child is naturally drawn to. Take note of these. Favorite activities and characters bring a feeling of excitement and joy to your child, and these positive feelings may help to alleviate discomforts in many different environments. We call these areas of preference your child's *preferred activities*. Preferred activities are simply the activities your child likes to do.

One of my students loves animals and insects. When books or videos contain animals and insects, he remains engaged for quite some time. We often observe how much he loves to line up the plastic animals, and then joyfully leap in circles, returning to view his animal lines again and again. For this child, this is a motivating preferred activity to work for and enjoy during his five-minute break from discrete trial learning. We also took our knowledge of this "preferred choice," and introduced this boy to mathematical patterns and beginning phonics patterns by putting those animal lines to work as manipulatives and as beginning sound (green animals) and ending sound (red animals) markers. And we introduced social lessons by using the animal lines to demonstrate following a group (walking in line), turn taking, waiting, and sharing.

When we are aware of a child's preferred activities, we have information about what may hold that child's interest, what may be reinforcing to that child, and where the child may show some better attending and self-regulating behaviors. *Preferred activities, even when seeming to be inappropriate fixations, can play an important role in the learning of social skills and concepts.* Favorite toys and characters can be used to help introduce and teach new ideas and lessons. They can also be used as motivators and rewards.

List here five of your child's preferred objects and activities:

1.

2.

3.

4.

5.

Nonpreferred Activities

I have a student who screams and bites his wrist when he sees the visual icon for "music class" on his "first-then" visual daily schedule. This child is a pleasure throughout most of the day, but he clearly does not prefer or enjoy the sounds and singing in the regular music class. Though adaptations were made for comfort's sake, we know this child would, if given the choice, prefer to be elsewhere, doing more personally enjoyable and stimulating things. Music, for him, is a *nonpreferred activity* owing to sensory sensitivities and uncomfortable experiences in the music environment.

Nonpreferred activities are the activities that children find undesirable, and the knowledge of a nonpreferred activity to come (even without being there) may set off behaviors that are not conducive to socializing. Children resist and avoid certain activities for many different reasons. These may include physical discomfort and sensory issues, skill level issues, or even separation and communication issues. When children show distinct aversions to certain kinds of activities, it is important to investigate *why* they are nonpreferred. This information is important and helpful when readying oneself and one's child to enter social situations. When we are aware of a child's nonpreferred activities, we have information about what disturbs the child, where and when his or her sensitivities really come to the forefront, and what to avoid—unless truly prepared for the child's resistant behaviors.

List here five of your child's nonpreferred objects and activities:

1.

2.

3.

4.

5.

Write down next to each entry what it is about these objects or activities that make them nonpreferred (if you know). Do they frustrate or scare your child in some way? Does your child possibly find a certain texture or environment uncomfortable? Your list will give you some information on your child's individual sensory and/or behavioral triggers.

Finding Age-Appropriate Interests

Finding friendship with same-age peers is difficult when developmentally a child does not share age-appropriate interests. And this is a common issue for children with autism. You should not feel pressured to limit your child's friendship possibilities and activities to same-age only. But do try to involve your child with others in his or her general age group. A general age group may be: preschool, lower elementary, higher elementary, middle school, or high school. I also recommend getting to know—through neighbors, friends, and family—the games, television shows, movies, and clothing typical children around your child's age are into. When children with autism are exposed to new movies, cartoons, or computer games, they often do show interest in the new motivating characters or toys. Perhaps a sibling close in age can help you identify these things (this is a great way to have siblings help their brother or sister), or possibly ask several neighborhood kids to help you "keep up with the times." Many kids would be happy to have the job of reporting back to you about changing peer interests, new shows, and "cool" movies to see.

Ultimately, we want all children, even kids with autism, to recognize conversational topics and have interests in common with others. I can't emphasize enough how the familiarity with current characters, movies, TV shows, and toys can help make the difference for many kids with autism, motivating them to stay and engage in, and even contribute to, conversations with peers. You *can* take your child to the movies (especially when using I.D.E.A.L.). You *can* teach your child what a Nintendo DS Lite is and introduce him to Bakugan toys.

Social Approachability

Your child's social approachability can determine whether peers will show interest in playing with or engaging with your child with autism. Try to look at your child as if you were seeing him through the eyes of others. How does your child with autism look? Is he clean, and wearing the same type of clothing the typical children wear? Is his hair in a style appropriate to his age? Is there an ABA specialist or aide with your child at all times with whom, together, they are their own island of private activity . . . or is the adult inviting other children in? And what do your child's behaviors look like from the outside? Do his facial expressions, movements, or unusual behaviors put children off? Or does your child attract other children?

Typical kids can be cautious, discriminating, and tough. They may notice and—not always kindly—comment on everything from a child's pant length, character lunchbox or backpack (especially when perceived as babyish), hairstyles, and more. They may make rude comments and joke about behaviors they perceive as unusual or weird.

Typical kids can also be very kind, intuitive, empathetic, and forgiving. In a group of typical kids, several often emerge as friends and helpers who can be trusted to have your child's best interests at heart. If your child is approachable, there will be children both typical and with special needs who will show a true desire to get to know your child for who he or she really is.

Several families that I work with have children with more severe autism. These kids struggle with intensive language difficulties as well as self-stimulating, self-injurious, and aggressive behaviors. They are not always socially approachable. Several of the autistic kids scare other children when in meltdown mode. But these same kids are also lovable and fun to be with much of the time, and peers get to see this side of them, too. When children with severe deficits are on track and self-regulated (with sensory outlets), they most certainly can join in on small-group social activities. They are supported and helped by both adults and peers to enjoy themselves, participate, and join in with friends. They even sometimes surprise us with their humor and unexpected contributions to the group!

It is important to work on social concepts and basic skills (which we will discuss very soon) to help children understand the rules of conversing and playing. But it is okay to get out into real-life environments before your child has the information down. It is okay for your child to do the "wrong" thing, and be corrected during real-life social activities and events. Wherever your child is at socially right now, this is the perfect starting point to progress from.

Teaching Social Concepts

Children with autism often need to be made aware of and taught (sometimes one small increment at a time) the simple interpersonal actions and expectations that most typical children simply pick up through observing family members, peers, and others in their environment. Some of the vocabulary may be new to you. If so, just keep in mind that, overall, we are simply talking about basic self-awareness and interpersonal skills.

Joint Attention

One of the first social skills that professionals would like to see children with autism demonstrate is joint attention. Joint attention involves sharing a moment with another, such as turning when one's name is called, making eye contact with another to share a laugh, or turning toward and listening to another person speak. Joint attention may also involve joining in on singing a song with a small group, or responding appropriately to a question. It requires an awareness of another (or others) and a clear attention to what is going on around one. A child may need to be prompted and then rewarded when showing joint attention. In a way, it really takes joint roles to make this skill successful. The teaching adults need to find what types of prompts bring the child to attention, and the child needs to decipher within himself how to bring his attention outward enough to receive a reward. Here are some simple ways to encourage joint attention that you can do in your home, during playdates, and during parties:

- Paint little pictures on the cheeks of your child and a playdate (hearts, flowers, logos, et cetera), and let them look at each other's faces as well as look at themselves in the mirror.

- Have your child pass out napkins, plates, or snacks to those he or she will be snacking with, and, if possible, have your child use a phrase such as "Here you go," or have your child ask a question such as "Do you want one or two?" so that the others can respond with a "thank you" or a quantity.

- Play a game such as "Get me the object I spy," where your child and others will listen to you (or a peer) describe an object in the room without naming it, and your child (and friends) will have to figure out and retrieve the object being "spied."

- Younger children may enjoy sitting on the floor or ground and rolling balls or trucks back and forth to each other.

One thing I have found with children with autism and joint attention is that children sometimes are attending along with a group but don't look as if they are. (Typical kids will tell you that they do the opposite—they look as if they are attending, but aren't really doing so.) For instance, a child with autism may be sitting with a class on a rug while a teacher reads a story, and the child with autism may be completely looking away from where the teacher is sitting and reading. It may look as if the child is not attending at all, but she may absolutely be listening. I have had to use prompts such as "*Show* you are listening" and "Turn your body, so he will know you are ready" so that the kids begin to learn and understand the unspoken expectations of the "look" of *joint* involvement.

Greeting

A skill that is also tackled early on is greeting another person. When greeting someone, a child must learn to briefly make eye contact and say "Hi." Later, a child may be expected to recognize and use the person's name in the greeting. For kids with autism, this may take a behind-the-scenes memorization task, in which they may learn and memorize names by looking at pictures of different people's faces. This technique may be used to help kids with autism learn the names of their classmates or extended family members so that they can later greet them. Often, a child with autism will need to be prompted to take notice of who is in the environment, but with practice and within a familiar environment, many children are able to perform this skill independently.

Upon greeting others, children with autism often get positively reinforced, by the responses and reactions of those they greet. Some kids with autism remember the names and faces of adults and peers from years earlier, and will continue to greet them in passing.

- It is helpful to begin greeting your child and prompting him or her to greet you back in your own home. When you walk into a room your child is in, or when your child comes to find you, say a simple "Hi" or "Hi" with a wave, and then tell your child to tell you "Hi" or "Hi, Mom," et cetera, back to you. Reduce your prompt after your child gets the hang of it, to a gesture or an "h" sound.

Play

Play is also a very important social skill, and there are many different levels of skills and expectations involved in play, many of which depend on children's ages. Children may begin with learning to play appropriately alongside others, and later advance to initiating play and joining into play that is already established. Learning appropriate play skills can be very challenging for children with autism. Kids who have more severe communicative issues and behaviors often do not understand the intent of the proximity of another—and may see it as an intrusion and react with anger. Some kids do not want their objects touched, so it is best to use some "neutral" toys and games when working on play skills with other kids. Preparing children beforehand for what is to come (which you will do as part of the I.D.E.A.L. process) will help to alleviate some of the stress for the children who need special help to play with others. As play skills are worked on, kids also learn to take turns (which involves joint attention), to share, to stop playing upon request (which is not always easy), and to clean up when asked or prompted.

- Be careful to choose toys and play environments that will not inflame your child's sensory sensitivities or rob her attention completely from her peers. For instance, your child may enjoy imaginative play, but when on a playdate, a peer may try to put the camping set's backpack onto your child's back, and may try to put the camping compass on your child's wrist. How will your child react?

- Some toys also have flashing lights and loud sounds. Some children with autism will avoid these toys and the kids using them, while others may become "obsessed" and fall into self-stimulation behaviors.

Communication

To sustain any social interaction, there must be communication between those who are involved. This could be verbal conversation, hand gestures, facial expressions, or sign language. Some children use communication boards or electronic devices to speak for them. Children with autism must learn when to make a communicative initiation or comment, and they must learn how and when to communicate a termination of an activity, as well as the need for help. They also must work on *self-awareness* so that they can recognize and communicate wants and needs through assessing their own moods or the signals they are receiving from their bodies (needing a break, needing to use the toilet, et cetera).

- Help your child to initiate a communication or conversation with others by helping him to approach and greet others.

- Help your child learn to comment by practicing "I like . . ." phrases and "I see . . ." phrases.

- Help your child learn to terminate an interaction by teaching him an ending phrase such as "See you later."

Perspective Taking

Perspective taking is a social skill that in generalized settings can be confusing for children with autism. Perspective taking involves seeing and understanding the emotions and/or viewpoints of others. Though children with autism may imitate emotion early on, they are often not aware of others' emotions, moods, or body language, and have to be taught incrementally what "happy" and "sad" are, as well as what they look like on other's faces. They must be taught through stories and examples how situations or events can make a person feel different emotions. Through practice, children may be able to identify the feelings of others by looking at their expressions or by understanding their situations. To help your child practice perspective taking skills:

- Cut out pictures of faces depicting different emotions from magazines, newspapers, or books. Have your child practice identifying the emotions on the faces of the people in the pictures. Try to describe to your child a time when he or she may have felt that emotion, or a time when you felt that emotion.

- As you read books to your child, or as your child reads to you, discuss the feelings of the characters and why they may feel like they do.

- Play with puppets and use the puppets to model and emphasize certain emotions. This is an activity your child can enjoy with peers, and peers can be pretaught which emotions or situations your child needs to work on.

Referencing

Another skill important for socialization is the ability to reference peers. Working toward independence is important for children with autism, and both parents and professionals do not want autistic kids learning to rely solely on their paraprofessionals' or teachers' prompts when functioning as part of a group. Referencing peers deals with looking around at others, or looking at a neighboring peer to see what she is doing, and then following suit. This is an important skill—especially for children who have difficulties with language processing. Children with language processing or attending difficulties are often unable to "catch" and process verbal direction. Referencing others allows for kids with autism to act appropriately—by taking visual cues from the environment. When a teacher tells a class to return to their desks, a student with autism may not process the direction before the commotion of movement toward the desks begins. But by referencing peers, a child with autism will be visually clued in, for the "language" of the movement of the class will communicate to that child what she should do. Here is a way to help your child practice referencing:

- Instead of taking your child's hand and leading him to the next location during an activity or event, prompt your child to "Look." (Or for more advanced children, you can say, "What should you be doing?") See if your child can discern where to go or what to do by looking at the others within the environment. Does your child see that all the other kids have lined up at the diving board (and then move to do the same)? Does your child see that everyone has moved to the table for cake? If not, you can gesture, and use simple phrases such as "You go, too," or "You do it, too."

In many social environments and activities, if a child with autism is confused, referencing a peer can help to get the child back on track. Of course, there will be those situations where you would rather your child *not* reference their peers—such as when kids are getting out of hand or rude—but this is typical of *all* kids. If you see this happen, redirect your child (and others), but don't forget to celebrate the referencing part!

Your child doesn't need to have all these skills down to be socially included. Even those who have little to no experience in social settings can begin to get more involved. So take heart. We want your child to, in the beginning, gain comfort so that she can self-regulate herself for a period of time among others. This will help to pave the way for building more advanced social skills and concepts later. You will get there—you just need to take one step at a time.

Your Child's Daily Rhythm and Activity Level

Socialization is so important for our children with autism that we must really look at and figure out which times of day each child is at his best. We want the children to be able to remember, be present, and find meaning in each social experience so that they can "lock away" that experience, and refer to it again. Children with autism can become very fatigued in school, therapy, and at home, especially if sleep is inconsistent. When looking at social activities and events, the time of day that an activity takes place will be a factor in the child's success. For some children, morning is when they are most attentive, while others may find a morning filled with sensory activities can help set up a productive afternoon. Each child has an individual daily rhythm that must be respected. We can help optimize a child's chance at success by determining the times of day a child may be most receptive to interacting with others. Children with autism also have natural mood fluctuations throughout the day, and natural ebbs and flows of their sensory sensitivities and tolerance throughout the day. And like the rest of us, a child with autism will naturally feel more irritable during certain periods of the day—possibly near mealtimes or after exerting themselves.

Take some notes or data for the next two days on your child's moods and availability for interacting with others. Use a Y for: Yes, good time to interact; and an N for: No, not a good time to interact. Every hour after waking (for instance, at 9 a.m., then at 10 a.m., et cetera), mark a Y or an N on a sheet of paper, and notice the times of day that may work well for playdates or activities. Notice which times of day to avoid.

Write down two different times of day your child is at his or her best:

1.

2.

Write down two different times of day it may be best to avoid social activities:

1.

2.

On the playground, and in many different social environments, typical children tend to gravitate toward other children who are engaging in activities and play in a way they find attractive. For instance, active boys tend to want to join boys who are playing actively. Your child's natural activity level will affect his interests, and attraction to being a participant in an activity. Your child's activity level will also affect which peers may be attracted to your child.

List three adjectives describing the type of play your child likes to engage in (active, quiet, musical, pretend, wet, messy, neat, artistic, mechanical, repetitive, indoor, outdoor, et cetera).

1.

2.

3.

The adjectives you have listed here will help you match your child's preferences to social and recreational activities we will discuss later in this book.

Verbal and Nonverbal Styles of Communication

Another consideration is your child's style of communication. Children with autism vary greatly in their language and intellectual abilities, and issues such as echolalia and delayed processing can make attempts at "conversing" with others very difficult. Some autistic children express themselves verbally and readily understand language that is said to them. Other kids are unable to speak, or simply do not have a grasp of basic language skills or concepts. Your child's verbal or nonverbal communication style will impact the type of preparation needed to help her be successful in social activities and events. It is important to be aware that even though your child may be able to use some words or sentences, she may process nonverbal, visual information more quickly. Every effort should be made to pair verbal communications with visual gestures, pictures, or other visual means to give the child the highest probability of understanding communication and of being understood. Some children with more severe issues use visual schedules, communication boards, picture exchange programs, and American Sign Language. When paired with simple language, these visual systems can *increase* the child's use of language and communicative initiations. Typical children are often fascinated by different types of communication, and want to know what they are and how they work. Knowing whether your child will need a system of communication other than or in addition to verbal communication is an important step in the planning and preparation for successful social involvement.

We will discuss this in more depth as we work with the I.D.E.A.L. system, but first let's take a close look at how our kids' sensory sensitivities and tolerance issues affect their socialization.

CHAPTER 2

■   ■   ■

Understanding Sensory Sensitivities
and Tolerance

She screams because she hates lifeguards. Not the people. The
whistle. It's loud. I don't like it either. Have you heard how loud
it is? It's loud. We hold our ears—like this. But mine don't hurt
as much as hers.

—LAINE, age six,
friend of Emma, who has pervasive developmental disorder–not otherwise
specified (PDD–NOS)

Imagine trying to act social, and remember rules, names, and
appropriate greetings, when the fluorescent gym lights are
emitting a sound that gives you that painful "nails on a chalk-
board" sensation, and you feel like you need to escape it or start
screaming. Children with autism often feel bombarded by the
sights and sounds in the environment, and their sensory processing difficulties can, at times, set off extreme reactions that we
find hard to understand. Sensitivities to noise, movement, or

touch can send kids into a tailspin behaviorally, which will often scare peers and cause family members and friends to leave activities prematurely—ruining social experiences for the entire family.

Sensory discomforts or the anticipation of them may cause many children with autism to experience extreme anxiety and to use whatever means possible, including negative behaviors, to try to avoid situations where these unwanted sensory experiences occur.

Sensory Processing in Social Environments

Children with autism may have worked for years refining skills and practicing phrases in ABA and therapeutic environments, but when they are in the presence of uncomfortable sensations and under stress, their chances of successfully using these skills largely decrease. Sensory processing of information in the environment—the sights, sounds, and bodily messages encountered in social activities—can truly be overwhelming. For parents and teachers, it is important to remember that, with all of us, a change in environment can mean a corresponding change in mood. Depending on our individual likes and dislikes and people preferences, a change in environment can mean a change in the way we regulate ourselves with others, or how much we attend to others. For children with autism, these differences can be profound.

When not prepared, autistic children can experience sudden change, and changes in environments, as shocks to their systems. The children seem to have a unique need for their bodies and minds to go through some sort of transitional adjustment when faced with change—something that may be hard for you and me to grasp. It is a shame seeing some of the children really faltering with skills because of bodily discomforts and needs—skills they may perform well in more conducive environments. This is why sensory processing issues need to be carefully considered *before* entering into social activities and new situations.

External and Internal Sensory Sensitivities and Tolerance

Most of the children with autism that I have worked with over the years have had clear *external sensory sensitivities*. This means that the children were extremely sensitive to experiences and stimuli originating from outside themselves. These would include lighting, sounds, movement, the feel of clothing, being touched, or visual stimuli in the environment around them. The sensory experiences the children feel internally, such as feeling the need to urinate, feeling dizzy with certain movements, feeling pain with incoming teeth, or feeling overwhelming emotion brewing, are called *internal sensory sensitivities*. Both external and internal sensory sensitivities can distract and overwhelm children with autism. The children should not be expected to handle and react to various situations in the way *we* would or their typical siblings would. We can, however, teach them appropriate ways— one step at a time—to handle uncomfortable situations as well as ways to remain as even and self-regulated as possible.

If we really look at when a child is overwhelmed, and begin to keep track of her discomforts, we can begin to differentiate between what is true misbehavior and what are needs that should be fulfilled. Also, by knowing and keeping track of your child's sensory sensitivities, you can make distinct choices for adaptations that will help her. We can prepare a child in advance, and give her brief, practice exposures to any uncomfortable elements. With more information, there is much that can be done. Information on an individual's sensory processing difficulties can help to shape preparation and define what can be expected within social events and activities. Knowing a child's sensory processing "mine fields" will, no doubt, help parents and teachers prepare in advance, so that the child's social experiences can be much more successful.

Seeking Behaviors in Social Situations

Jack has autism, but he most certainly wants contact, and seeks out both people and objects to hug and squeeze. He can truly be lovable and adorable, but there are days when he is so in need of tight contact and pressure that he hugs, squeezes, scratches, and butts heads to desperately get a feeling he is seeking. Sometimes he is irritable and will try to throw himself against us to get immediate and deep sensory input. Being held tight with hugs or squeezes is calming and organizing for Jack.

Early on, Jack was able to show us through his actions what he needed, and by observing the types of contact he sought, we could take note of what had positive effects on his demeanor. His initiations for contact, though, were for the most part, not appropriate. Even though Jack could use some words and very simple phrases appropriately, he would not use his language when seeking sensory fixes. His sensory needs would literally overtake him. Because the resulting feeling of hugs and squeezes are so positive and motivating for Jack, he is now being taught to use simple language to request what he needs. He will now say, "Hug, please," or "Squeeze, please." (Kids without language may be able to gesture, or hand over a picture card depicting a "hug.")

Socialization can be very difficult for children who seek sensory stimulation because of the way their seeking behaviors appear in the midst of peers. Children with autism do not tend to socially edit their words or actions, and typical children do take notice when children lick and bite toys or play in an aggressive fashion that causes unwelcome contact.

Parents often ask me questions regarding whether they should speak with typical peers about their child's atypical behaviors, and I do believe it is helpful to be honest with typical kids. You can be informative, but not too personal, if you talk with them in a simple and age-appropriate way. Typical children, when educated and told the truth—for instance, if they are told a certain child does not understand how to approach others appropriately but is learning—will often rise to the occasion and help in ways adults cannot. Typical children can engage other children, whether typical or with special needs, in ways adults cannot. Children with autism have peers, and are peers, and children need to learn to function and play among their peers. Differences in children allow for learning opportunities for all children.

Parents can help diminish seeking behaviors in social situations by providing sensory fixes before the activity or event. You can also bring "a bag of tricks" to provide sensory input that will help your child self-regulate herself better, leading to a more appropriate demeanor. We will discuss these in more detail later in this chapter.

Avoidance Behaviors in Social Situations

Joseph doesn't like to be touched, and is bothered by the close proximity of other children. He also does not like his preferred objects to be touched, moved, or talked about if the "talk" disturbs the self-talk that he engages in. He tries to avoid sitting next to other children and adults, and will scream with a high-pitch whine if he is touched. Joseph has language—he will say "Can you go away?" often and will sometimes accompany this request with a shove. Not too conducive for socializing. But Joseph is dealing with a very difficult sensory processing issue called *tactile defensiveness*, which makes him do his best to avoid what he perceives as pain or discomfort when touched. Like seeking behaviors, avoidance behaviors can become more aggressive if the child feels the need to avoid the unwanted discomfort at all costs.

Avoidance behaviors initially need to be addressed by the adults in the child's environment, because a child with autism who is trying to avoid a situation is usually not "available" for reasoning, thinking before acting, or making good choices while needing to escape. This is why it is so important to know the child's sensory triggers, and to keep track (data) of when they occur and the stimuli they are in response to. Remember, every child is truly individual from another. Autism shows itself uniquely in each child. Adaptations, as part of the I.D.E.A.L. process, can make huge differences for children who act inappropriately when trying to avoid and escape uncomfortable stimuli.

Becoming aware of a child's seeking or avoidance behaviors (some children may have both) can help us prepare them for what they may encounter in different social activities and in varied environments. Both the seeking and avoiding of sensory stimulation, whether external or internal, can disrupt and impede an autistic child's ability to attend to and process what is going on and being said around them. Preparing so that sensory seeking will be reduced, and so that the need to avoid certain stimuli will not be as apparent or necessary, can help a child be more available for the experience and enjoyment of relating to others.

Increasing Sensory Tolerance

With your help (and in many cases, with the help of occupational therapy), children with autism can increase their sensory tolerance. This means that they can learn to better tolerate and cope with the internal and external discomforts that distract them. Professionals often call this *sensory desensitization*. Sensory desensitization takes time and patience. Children are exposed to small doses of the unwanted stimuli for tiny increments of time. In the beginning, this would be done indirectly, but with time, the child could be exposed more directly to the stimuli. Here is an example:

> Bryce is scared to walk on the sidewalk to the right of his house because the neighbors have a dog. He will also refuse to go outside in his backyard when the dog is out in the neighbor's yard. The dog is a friendly family pet, and both Bryce's parents and the neighbors have tried numerous times to introduce the two in a calm, nonthreatening way,

but Bryce has fought, scratched, and bitten to remain far away. This hasn't always been a major issue, but recently Bryce started to refuse to go to his bus, and his behavior, both coming and going from his school bus, has affected his reputation with the neighborhood kids, who see his meltdowns on a daily basis. Bryce's parents are upset that the kids see him at his worst. Also, the neighbors feel unintentional pressure to keep their dog in during "bus times" and after school, so that Bryce can go outside and not feel afraid. Bryce's mother mentioned that grandparents and family friends have to confine their pets in separate rooms or basements when they, on rare occasions, visit.

The goal is not for Bryce to have direct contact with the dog—but to be able to tolerate the dog—possibly even ignore the dog. To help begin to desensitize Bryce, we gave him some indirect contact with the dog, by video recording the dog with his sister, Emma. She had been instructed to play by herself near the dog, and to ignore the dog. If the dog beckoned for attention, she was instructed to say, "Hi, Noodle" (and she could give the dog a quick pet), and then return to her play. Bryce was fascinated by this DVD, and watched it repeatedly.

Next, Bryce's mother put a chair on the back patio (when the dog was out back), right against the glass sliding door into the house, and announced she would be handing out fruit snacks (a favorite of Bryce's). Bryce was not allowed to eat his fruit snacks inside, nor in the doorway to his backyard. He had to sit in the chair designated by his mom. If he began to tantrum or whine, his mother would turn and walk away with the fruit snacks. Bryce finally agreed, and began to eat his snack in the chair on the patio.

Emma was then instructed to go play in the proximity of the dog as she did on the DVD. Watching Emma from the patio chair was not as fear invoking, because Bryce had already been introduced to the scenario via the previously filmed DVD. Over time, Bryce became more desensitized, and was able to self-regulate much better in the presence of this dog.

Bryce's parents use similar previewing techniques for other new experiences, since he tends to be overly sensitive, and the previewing helps him maintain more appropriate behaviors and responses.

Simple Sensory Solutions

Children who seek sensory "input" are trying to fulfill a need. Supplying objects or exercises that fulfill this need can help a child self-regulate for a duration of time. Sometimes sensory solutions are as simple and logical as carrying a small portable set of headphones for loud environments. It is important to anticipate and prepare for sensory and tolerance difficulties, as well as learn ways to gracefully handle unwanted sensory "surprises."

The *tactile* sense, and the lesser known *proprioceptive* and *vestibular* senses, play important roles in most of our daily tasks and actions. When not functioning properly in a child, or when a child's brain does not make sense of the information properly (sensory integration dysfunction), children often react in ways that seem extreme or in ways that are hard to understand. Some children exhibit atypical or inappropriate responses.

The tactile sense receives sensations through our skin. Your child will react to touch sensations according to his or her perception and integration of the tactile information. What some kids feel as a tickle, others will feel as pain. Your child's peers need to be alerted in social situations if your child does not like to be touched.

The proprioceptive sense gathers information from our muscles, tendons, ligaments, and skin, and tells us where our limbs are, what our body position is, and how to grade—use our judgment to control, aim, or manage—our motions. With our proprioceptive sense, we can anticipate how much force we need to put a key into a lock, to open a door, to set one foot in front of the other, as well as how much force to use when hugging another. Proprioception that is dysfunctional may turn a friendly hug into what may feel like an aggressive hold. During playdates or social activities, parents can use verbal and gestural cues to help their children keep track of and adjust, if necessary, their actions, as they learn to gain awareness about the proper amounts of force or motion required for different actions.

The vestibular sense gives us information about our body orientation—in essence, where we are in relation to gravity. Vestibular sensors are tucked deep in our inner ears, and help us to remain upright and balanced. Children often have highly sensitive vestibular senses, so great care should be taken with activities that include spinning, flipping, or motions that can affect one's equilibrium.

Sensory processing issues are a hallmark of autism, and most children with an ASD filter environmental and bodily information either too intensely or not enough. Some children are considered to be *hypersensitive*, meaning they may be overly reactive to stimuli, while others are *hyposensitive*, and are unusually underreactive or nonreactive to stimuli in and around them. A young student I used to work with, Cassie, used to spend up to ten minutes rubbing the place on her arm or shoulder that accidentally brushed a classmate in the hallway, as if she could not get the sensation off her arm. She clearly had tactile hypersensitivity. A young boy I evaluated named Jacob didn't know when he needed to use the toilet, that is, until he felt the sensation of going on his outer skin. He also would not stop eating unless portions were controlled, because no matter how much he would eat, he would not feel full. Jacob was hyposensitive to important bodily sensations, and this caused him to have "accidents" and to vomit at times. It is not uncommon to have a child with mixed sensitivities, where the child may be hypersensitive to sounds and tastes yet hyposensitive to bodily sensations, like Jacob was.

A child's sensory processing and individual ability or inability to filter environmental and bodily information greatly influence her state of *arousal*. If a child's state of arousal becomes high through an active or highly stimulating activity, she may need assistance reducing her state of arousal through calming tasks or through physical removal to a place that will help to calm her down. A child who is overly aroused may become behaviorally difficult, or shut down completely. You may hear child professionals call this *sensory overload*, and this state of being overwhelmed is very uncomfortable for the child. It is important to know that children with autism have a difficult time reducing their own states of arousal, and may truly need some verbal, gestural, or visual guidance to return to a more regulated and calmer state. Reducing stimuli in the environment, or moving to a quiet area, may be helpful, as well as using visual charts that depict calming strategies—such as sitting and counting to 10.

Many parents have found that deep pressure has a profound effect on their kids' moods and self-regulation. This is often given in ball "squishes" and comforter "wrap-ups." (For more information on deep pressure interventions, please speak with an occupational therapist.) Many children with autism also love being rubbed with different textures, for they find it calming and soothing.

By gaining an awareness of the sensory difficulties that are unique to your child, you can have preplanned "escapes" and sensory "fixes" that will help your child remain self-regulated for longer periods of time; and that will help your child *regain* self-regulation in the moments following an overload from the stimuli or activity around her.

Let's do a simple exercise that will help you highlight your individual child's sensory and tolerance trouble spots, as well as the environmental "red flags" that may set off his undesirable behaviors. Write your answers in the space provided or use a separate piece of paper if necessary:

My child gets excited when _____

_____.
(What is the predominant sense your child is using when excited?)

My child gets scared when _____

_____.
(What is the predominant sense your child is using when scared?)

My child likes to be touched in the following ways:
(Next to each entry below, state whether that particular touch calms or arouses your child.)

1.

2.

3.

My child does not like to be touched in the following ways:
(Next to each entry below, state what he does to avoid or stop these types of touches.)

1.

2.

3.

How does your child react to the following sensory experiences?
(Note: Your child may have different reactions to, for instance, soft sounds or music as opposed to loud sounds—please note these differences.)

1. Sound: _____

_____

_____

2. Lights: _____

_____

_____

3. Voices: _____

_____

_____

4. Motion (such as swinging): _____

_____

_____

5. Heat: _____

_____

_____

6. Cold: _____

_____

_____

7. Commotion or action: _____

_____

_____

8. Eating: _____

_____

_____

9. Pain: _____

_____

_____

10. Wearing clothing: _____

_____

_____

11. Bathing: _____

_____

_____

12. Tooth brushing, hair brushing: _____

_____

_____

13. Toileting: _____

_____

_____

14. Hugging: _____

_____

_____

15. Riding in a car: _____

_____

_____

16. Animals: _____

_____

_____

17. Storms: _____

_____   _____

_____

By doing this simple exercise, you may already see a pattern emerging that points to your child's individual sensory "hot spots," but pattern or no pattern, the information you have gathered will be invaluable as we use I.D.E.A.L. to prepare for and accommodate your child's sensitivities and needs, so that he can more successfully participate in social activities.

First, let's take a look at the nonconducive behaviors and safety issues that can arise from high arousal levels, sensory processing issues, and communication deficits as our children with autism try to join in and participate with others.

CHAPTER 3

■　■　■

Nonconducive Behaviors and Safety

We don't go to the mall and we can't go to anything outside, or a place that has lots of doors, because my brother bolts. You have to hold on to him and sometimes he kicks me and I can't hold on, and I'm totally scared he'll run into a street or something and get hit by a car.

—SHANNON, *age eight,*

big sister to Riley, who has autism with mental retardation

Children with autism are often unaware of dangers around them or the possible negative consequences of quick, impulsive actions or behaviors. And for their parents, fears about the implications of a single "wrong move" on their child's part have kept many families from venturing away from the safety of their home and school environments.

"He's a fast kid," one mother told me, "and I just don't know if I would be able to stop him in time if he should run off. I would never forgive myself, you know, if something happened."

Sadly, as with this mom of an autistic third-grader, the resulting isolation takes a toll on all members of the family, and does not help the child learn more appropriate coping and adaptive skills.

Parents often find difficult, dangerous, or aggressive behaviors hard to handle in the home, so even just thinking of dealing with the same behaviors out in public domains feels beyond overwhelming to them. It is very hard for a family to teach appropriate behavior and not reinforce (even accidentally) inappropriate behavior when major safety issues arise, or when outside persons act disturbed at what they are seeing and involve themselves.

Worries about the safety of their child, the safety of other children, and concerns about maintaining their child's dignity (and their own dignity) in difficult situations, have caused parents to back away from many activities. A lot of parents feel their child would encounter just too many dangers and too many unknowns. Fears and hesitancy, for many parents of children with autism, are like constant companions that must be confronted head on, over and over again. But even a little bit of new knowledge can help decrease difficult behaviors. And learning to plan ahead can help skirt unwanted situations.

One way to prevent undesirable behaviors is to engage your child in activities that are incompatible with their inappropriate behaviors.

One simple example of this would be the child who bites other children when anxious. Providing a hard candy or lollipop for the child to suck, or having the child eat fruit snacks while sitting or waiting, can help him self-regulate better. The idea is to engage the child's mouth (if he bites) or hands (if she grabs or hits) in appropriate ways when entering into anxiety-producing situations. This way, the undesirable actions are *incompatible* with what the child is doing.

Addressing a Lack of Interest and Lack of Engagement

Children with or without autism tend to regulate their moods less in situations that hold no interest for them. All children co-operate and participate more in social activities when "something is in it for them." For some children, the positive attention of others may be reinforcing in itself. On the other hand, some kids get lots of social attention fast by misbehaving. Because entering any new situation can be difficult for an autistic child, it is important to choose activities carefully, and to help your child prepare for the unknown. In essence, you will be trying to make the unknown *known* before actually attending an activity or event. I will show you how to do this in Chapter Six.

So how is it that we get a child to enter a situation that may be uncomfortable? The way we begin to do this is by introducing an activity, and then pairing the activity with known and preferred objects and activities. It will be helpful if you look back at the information you have gathered (from Chapter One) on your individual child's preferred activities. Let's take the example of a child who likes cheese puffs. The act of eating cheese puffs may be enjoyable and familiar. Pairing this with the new situation of attending a birthday party, where the child may eat cheese puffs in the proximity of other children at the party, can begin a pathway to further comfort and interaction at birthday parties and other similar activities. Of course, this situation may be more suitable to a child whose autistic symptoms are more severe, but children with higher-level abilities also greatly benefit from preparation, and the comforting presence of familiar objects or activities in new situations and surroundings.

I have witnessed many a therapist and teacher throw their hands up and give up when a child with autism does not attend to them or appear to have interest in the activities or initiated interactions of those around them. Sometimes children with autism, like all children, are simply not interested in or motivated by a subject matter or activity. Also, from my own work with the children, I know that even when the subjects at hand are not the going favorites, the children with autism are still positively affected by the *familiarity* of the people they are with, and the familiarity of the surroundings. They show an increased attention and engagement in activities when this comfort level is present.

What this means is that in the realm of socialization and social activities and events, success may not come on the first outing. The children may need to show up repeatedly, even for small increments of time, to establish more comfort. The increased comfort will allow for greater attention, participation, and ease with those around them.

In a way, I see children with autism slowly expanding an imaginary circle around themselves. In each new situation, they are very self-distracted and self-absorbed with the new sensations of the new situation. After comfort emerges in their sensory selves, the children begin to slowly attend out from themselves more than initially. Even if they only want to be in a certain area, or are impulsively exploring or pacing the perimeter, they begin to form a wider mental picture of themselves within the space. If repeated exposure allows for their comfort to grow, the kids will begin to notice and gain awareness of the entire environment and the people within the environment.

Curbing Aggressive Behaviors and Tantrums

Children are not accepted socially when their peers (and/or parents) are simply afraid of them or uncomfortable being around them. And in both school and recreational environments, children do remember and talk about peers who tantrum, hurt, or behave differently than others. Children also take a lot of cues from the adults in their environments and *their* reactions in difficult situations. This is why it is important to be honest and up-front (in a matter-of-fact way) about behaviors that may appear in a social situation. It always amazes me how helpful, when informed about what to expect, both children and adults are— even those who know very little about autism and behavior. Children, like all of us, are different people, and will have different reactions and questions about situations that arise. And while some parents would rather not have to discuss their child's disability with other children, I would recommend that it be done. For children with higher-functioning autism, this may not be needed.

When preparing to work on behavior, it is important to begin a little note taking behind the scenes, such as keeping track of when, where, and why tantrums and aggression are occurring. This is where "data" comes into the picture, but don't let the word "data" scare you. You simply want to record the times of day the behaviors are occurring, and what the "meltdowns" were in reaction to. Also, record what was done in response, because often children with autism learn unwanted lessons. For instance, if you hug your child tightly when he begins punching you (you may hug tight to stop the punching and to calm your child), your child may learn that when he feels agitated or uncomfortable, he should begin punching to get quick and calming help (the tight hug). Another example would be, if your child begins screaming in a mall and you give him crackers to quiet him, he may learn that when he feels the need for something in his mouth, or something to eat (or feels discomfort), he should scream to be given a comforting object or food. So, even though the last thing you may want to do is write down these things in the turmoil and aftermath of a tantrum or aggressive episode, the information will truly be important for seeing patterns.

Tantrums and aggression are often related to frustrations surrounding communication, and sensory issues that make self-regulation challenging. From your mood recordings in Chapter One, you may already be aware of daytime "hot spots," and from Chapter Two, sensory "hot spots," so you may be able to pinpoint certain times and factors that make your child more "available" to socially interact. You may have also found that certain times of the day or evening may be better weathered in the comfort of your home.

Once you have more information on why certain behaviors are occurring (transitioning, not getting what she wants when she wants it, avoidance, et cetera), you can begin to make a plan of preventative steps to reduce the need for the aggressive behaviors and tantrums.

But again, this is easier said than done. It is not always easy to decipher why certain aggressive behaviors occur. And what the child communicates with the behavior may not always be the same.

One child I work with is quick to anger—especially when told "no." But we can lower his arousal level through sensory input breaks, so when he becomes angry, his behavior is *less* aggressive and violent owing to his body's needs having been previously met. When his sensory breaks are missed, his anger is at a heightened, hard-to-control level because his arousal levels have not been relieved.

For several of the students I work with, a "quiet area" or "safe area" works well to reduce the early signs of stress or agitation. A quiet area can be as simple as a chair placed in a quiet corner of a room, or can be a small room that has very little stimuli in it. It is a place to relax without demands. Children who are stressed and aroused can spend a few minutes (the amount of time is very individual for each child) in a quiet area to regain self-regulation or clear thinking. Sensory tools can be incorporated into quiet areas for true relief from agitating situations.

When a child is aggressive in social situations (and a child can become aggressive if overly hungry, confused, frustrated, uncomfortable, or *when he does not know what to expect or does not understand what is going on*), the arousal level of the child will need to be reduced, but we do not want to reward the child by handing him something preferred as a calming agent. First, and foremost, it is important that if the possibility of aggression is present in a social situation, we want to have the preplanning for it that will ensure the safety of all.

If you expect that your child's arousal level may be heightened in social settings, here are a few things you can do to try and preempt a tantrum:

- Give your child calming sensory input or gross motor exercise before an activity.

- Bring your child to a quiet "safe area."

- Use your child's known form of communication as well as additional visuals to reduce confusion.

- Reduce lighting, or noise if possible, or reduce or move your child away from other sensory inputs (people standing too close or touching your child).

- Give the child a snack or drink.

- Don't ask more of your child than he or she can handle on that particular day.

Sometimes little things go a long way. Giving your child tight hugs (while behaving nicely) and squeezes can provide some deep pressure that may reduce the sensory-seeking behaviors that can, when aroused, manifest as charging, crashing, or punching. A couple fruit snacks to chew twice an hour may reduce oral sensory-seeking behaviors that may manifest as biting when agitated. If and when possible, help by reducing sound, commotion, or visual stimuli (fewer objects and less color) to help keep arousal and agitation levels down. All of these can help a child remain better regulated so that he will be more available for more appropriate forms of communication.

But sometimes your child may launch himself into a full-blown tantrum, and here are a few things you can do to weather it:

- Reduce the amount of language you are using with your child, and try not to ask questions. Use short, declarative statements. For example, don't say, "Stop it right now! Do you want some water?" Instead, try, "Shhh. Here's water."

- Use statements such as, "I will help. You want . . ." (See if your child can finish the statement with words, a visual, or device.)

- Use statements naming a preferred object, activity, or need, such as, "You sit, then get a squish." (For some children, do use the question form: "Want squish? Then sit.")

- If your child acts out with hitting, throwing, or other more aggressive behaviors, clearly and strongly state, "No hitting. You sit." Or "No biting. Use your words."

I worked with a young boy who, upon losing control, would run at me to punch, but I would strongly say, "Arms down. Use your words." And (halfway to me) he would.

You may also find in some cases that your child is using tantrum behaviors and aggression to get your attention. If your child is not in danger, you may need to ignore these behaviors. When your child is calm, teach her to use words or a gentle touch. Take her hand and have her touch you, say or sign "Mom," and look at her in anticipation. Do it again and again if you have to, and once she gets the idea, say "Yes, [your child's name]" and immediately give her your full attention, or immediately get her communication board and give her your full attention. This is, of course, just one example, but *you want your child to learn that she will get what she needs by doing a very simple and appropriate action—one that is simpler than a tantrum or an aggressive behavior.*

The Nitty-Gritty of Working on Behavior

There are two types of behavior we commonly work on with our kids:

- Behavior we would like to see more of, and therefore *increase*

- Behavior we would like to see less of, and therefore *decrease*

You have the power to arrange consequences so that your children will learn that something is in it for them to react differently and possibly substitute or change their behavioral habits. Behaviors we would like to increase usually include polite behavior, attending, appropriate affectionate behavior, and appropriate play. Behaviors we would like to decrease include aggression, tantrums, and inappropriate self-stimulation behaviors.

There are specific behavioral interventions you can use to achieve each of these.

To arrange consequences for *behaviors you would like to increase*, use *reinforcements* or *reinforcers*. Did you know that something is only reinforcing when it increases the behavior? Reinforcers are given to a child only after performing the "target" behavior. (You may hear professionals say, "Reinforcers are *contingent* upon the performance of a target behavior.")

The most common type of reinforcement is *positive reinforcement*, and positive reinforcers must be something meaningful to the child, or something the child wants or enjoys. So, positive reinforcers can be hugs, high-fives, candy and other edibles, a favorite toy, or a tickle.

Sometimes positive reinforcers are given immediately after a target behavior occurs, but when a child begins to perform the behavior often, to receive the reinforcers, we can form a *schedule of reinforcement*, where the child may have to perform the behavior three times in a row to get the reinforcer (and many use visuals or tokens for the child to see and understand this). Some may move to *intermittent reinforcers*, where the child is rewarded only intermittently—so the child continues to perform the target behavior hoping to be rewarded—but not knowing exactly when the reward will come.

Another type of reinforcement is *negative reinforcement*. Negative reinforcement also increases wanted behavior, by removing a preferred object or activity until the expected target behavior is performed. Children in schools often encounter negative reinforcement such as losing recess when their work is not finished in the time allotted. Many children will increase their on-task behavior (the target behavior the teacher wants to increase) to avoid missing recess.

To arrange consequences for *behaviors you would like to decrease*, you can use several different techniques.

Many professionals like to use *differential reinforcement*. Differential reinforcement works by reinforcing lower rates of the target behavior, reinforcing the nonoccurrence of a behavior, or reinforcing incompatible behaviors.

When we choose to reinforce lower rates of behavior (DRL), we positively reinforce the child when he does not perform the target behavior (remember, the behavior we want to decrease) within an interval of time, or when the child shows a reduction of the target behavior within a time interval—which, for example, could be every five minutes, every half hour, et cetera. To do this properly, we would take some data to see how many times the child is performing the behavior we want to decrease. Let's say your child screeches ten times within a fifteen-minute time period. You could set up a schedule of reinforcement where your child would only be reinforced every fifteen minutes if he screeches no more than six times. Once your child is able to decrease to that level, you could either change the time interval to reflect the progress, or expect your child to decrease the screeching to only three times within the fifteen-minute time interval.

Sometimes reinforcement will be given to a child only if the targeted behavior *does not occur at all* during a time interval. This is called *differential reinforcement of other behavior* (DRO). If a child performs the targeted behavior even once, the time interval will be restarted immediately.

A DRO schedule of reinforcement worked well for an autistic student I worked with one summer. This young boy would grind his teeth almost constantly. His teeth grinding was loud and would elicit very negative reactions from both adults and other students in his proximity (and was ruining his teeth). We began with two-minute intervals of the expected behavior of "quiet mouth." Expectations were explained in advance through a "social story." A timer would be set for the two-minute interval, and if he did not grind during the interval, he received one pizza-flavored cracker (a highly preferred snack food). The pizza cracker motivated this boy to remain aware and to try to control the grinding, and the frequent chewing of the cracker helped him to physically keep a better check on his mouth. At times, he did begin to grind, and in these instances, we would reset the timer for a new interval. We were able to extend the intervals to eight minutes in the sixth week of this DRO program.

Schedules of reinforcement can also be set up to reinforce incompatible behaviors, and this is done by guiding children to activities that are incompatible with their unwanted behaviors. *Differential reinforcement of incompatible behaviors* (DRI) reinforces a child for his participation in appropriate activities that cannot coincide with the target *unwanted* behavior. If the child scratches and pinches, the use of hand-held squishy balls, rubber bands, pieces of tape, fine motor toys, or other objects that the child can manipulate with his hands can help the child to refrain from other inappropriate uses of his or her hands and refrain from inappropriate actions. The child can earn reinforcements and rewards for appropriate behavior.

Some other behavioral techniques to decrease behavior include:

- Extinction

- Response cost

- Time-outs

Extinction usually means ignoring unwanted behavior, and this can take some time to work. The idea is that you are giving the unwanted behavior absolutely no reinforcement whatsoever, and because in the child's eyes, they may at first be unsure why their "tried and true" behaviors are no longer working—you may see an increase in the behavior initially because the child will try to use what has worked before to a more intense and possibly louder degree. If you can make it through the increase, the child will learn that the behavior is no longer working, which will show in time as a decrease or complete extinction of the behavior.

Response cost is considered to be a form of punishment, because if an unwanted behavior occurs, a desirable item or activity is taken away. Many use the response cost strategy with a token system, where the child will be earning tokens toward a wanted reinforcer, and if a behavioral misstep occurs, a token will be taken away. Sometimes an undesirable bout of behavior may cost children their privileges to a favorite toy, the computer, or TV.

Time-outs are frequently used to reduce unwanted behavior in children, but few know that in addition to being separated, the main idea behind "time out" is to be *without any reinforcement* for a designated time period—no matter what the behavior during the time period. A child should move to or be guided to a specific area designated for the time-out, and not spoken to until the time period has ended. Many use the time guideline of one minute per year of age for children, but children with autism may need this to be reduced because of developmental immaturity.

No matter which behavioral strategies you choose to decrease unwanted behavior, it is important to simultaneously teach your child more appropriate substitutions, or *replacement behaviors.* Model the behavior you would like your child to use instead, and prompt her to imitate you. Make sure to positively reinforce all efforts your child makes to perform the replacement behaviors.

How to Handle Bolting

If your child bolts, this can be a major safety concern, and even if it happens rarely, this behavior needs to be taken seriously, and be preventatively planned for. Children with autism bolt from their caregivers for many reasons. Some of these may include pure avoidance, a true want to return to or find a preferred place or activity, or some kids just bolt for the sheer joy of being chased—which can be very stimulating. Even children who have bolted on only one occasion may end up excluded from participation in activities in natural settings owing to safety fears.

The steps in I.D.E.A.L. will help you decrease the possibility of bolting from occurring. Children with autism who bolt are not all alike, so the reactions within certain environments, the sensory issues, and the reasons for running off will be different. Understanding the "whys" of your child's bolting will help a lot in prevention. Strategic placement of adults can be helpful, so you may want to ask friends or recreational leaders for their assistance in creating multiple shadows for your child in recreational environments if he is a bolter. Using visuals as well for stress-free communication methods and reinforcement systems (you want something the child can readily, even immediately understand) can help, too.

Behind the scenes, in your home, begin to work on responding appropriately to the word "stop." Each time your child appropriately stops in reaction to your demand, reward your child. You may need to model the behavior for your child first if she does not understand what is expected, or you may be able to have a sibling model the behavior of "stopping" when an adult says, "Stop." Use a picture symbol for "stop" and pair it with the verbal demand, if needed for further understanding.

If you use a system at home or in the child's school environment that helps to reduce the child's bolting, you may want to use some of the same symbols or methods in a recreational environment. Some of the children I have worked with have responded to stop signs on doors or visuals depicting a loss of reinforcement. We have also placed X's on the floor in red or yellow thick tape. The kids that would bolt during transitions to nonpreferred activities would not be verbally told to go to these nonpreferred areas. Simply hearing the words would send them off and running. Instead, they would be directed to go to an X, where they would be positively reinforced. They would then be directed to a distinct marker or chair within the nonpreferred location—where they would then be reinforced for standing or sitting at the correct marker.

Bolting can also be controlled by using *active patterns*. Active patterns are particularly helpful when bolting is related to transitioning issues. Active patterns can be familiar songs, footsteps, or hand motions set to "sing-songy" auditory patterns—which you repeat over and over again until you reach your destination. For instance, one active pattern may be: *1 . . . 2 . . . 3 . . . Slap!* (You slap hands together or give a high-five to each other.) This pattern would be repeated verbally with the motions over and over again until reaching the new location safely. Children with autism enjoy active patterns and may truly like singing the chorus to their favorite song over and over again with a little jump, turn, or handshake embedded just for fun.

Handling Sensory Defensiveness

It can be hard enough when your child isn't showing interest in other children, or isn't initiating interactions appropriately, but when this is coupled with your child's recoiling from the presence of other children, or the possible close proximity of or touch of a peer, socialization becomes much more difficult. Sensory processing difficulties, including tactile defensiveness, can be improved with the help of *sensory diets* (tactile, vestibular, and proprioceptive activities and therapies), which are overseen by occupational therapists. But as your child works to increase his sensory tolerance, you should let others know that he does not like to be touched. You can tell adults as well as younger children that your child feels "touches" differently than we do. Both adults and children find this knowledge fascinating, and can adjust their own behaviors to make interacting more comfortable for your child.

Working with Physical Difficulties

If your child's issues are more pervasive and include fine and gross motor difficulties, oral motor issues, or other physical issues, these will need to be considered when choosing activities and outings to attend. I will teach you to do this as part of the I.D.E.A.L. process. It is important to choose an activity for your child that will highlight a strength she has. It is also important to consider whether your child can participate in a way that will allow for some positive interactions with peers. This can get a little tricky in some activities. For example, children with gross motor difficulties may not be at their best in team sports, but there may be some terrific neighborhood kids that interact with your child and may be thrilled to help your child participate. I know of several instances where the coaches and teammates were helpful and willing to include children with autism with and without physical difficulties. But I also know of a situation where a certain soccer team did well, and began to play championship games. In the team's successful progression forward, the attitudes of the autistic child's teammates changed— they felt it was unfair to have him come on the field for his typical chunk of playing time. It is sad that this situation arose, making it hard to keep the social aspect of this child's participation positive. So, I want to mention that these issues come up, and can be looked at from many different perspectives. Winning, achieving, personal rewards, and sportsmanship mean different things to different people, including children. Though typical children do not understand the experience of autism, they do understand working hard to achieve—so be ready for some thought-provoking situations. All children should have the right to participate. Expect some give, and take, but also model give-and-take. There are some good lessons for all of us in each new situation.

Dealing with Foods, Medications, and Special Diets

As parents become more aware of the different avenues of treatment for autism, and the possibility of both special diets and medications helping to alleviate some of the difficult symptoms, they are finding that additional preparation needs to be taken before attending social events and activities so that their children will not be thrown off course by eating undesirable foods, or by missing scheduled doses of medication. Though it may be difficult to hold some kids back from cupcakes or cookies that are not gluten- or casein-free, parents should arrive at an event armed with attractive food alternatives, and know beforehand when or if food will be out or included as part of an activity. Sometimes children with autism truly have food preferences and would much rather snack on or celebrate with favorites brought from home. Also, medication delivery should be considered. Parents need to know how and where they could deliver medication to their child without disturbing their child's positive participation in an activity or event. For any foods or medications that may need refrigeration, parents should call beforehand to see if there is an accessible refrigerator, or plan to bring a cooler. Some children with autism need to drink water or juice often, and having these familiar drinks handy can help kids to maintain positive moods.

Sharing Responsibility for Safety

Parents do not have to tackle their children's socialization experiences alone. To help make social events and activities successful for children with autism, it is important for parents to be very upfront with activity leaders and family about issues and behaviors that may come up during activities or events. When given the knowledge of safety concerns, most persons involved really help by troubleshooting with you ways to ensure safe participation. Whether this involves modifying an activity, or strategically using people to block doorways or to create safer boundaries, the sharing of responsibility for the children's safety can be both rewarding and informative to all. Parents' information on their child combined with others' knowledge of the environments can make for very successful outings so never hesitate to speak up or ask questions. Many activity leaders have never had a child with autism in their groups (this will promptly change), but are absolutely willing and excited to have special kids in their activities. Perhaps some family members have never had the chance to help your child enjoy a special holiday, but would love the opportunity to do so. Not all initial attempts work out perfectly, but what is learned from those first attempts is invaluable to making subsequent social outings and events successful.

We will look further at enlisting help from parents, teachers, and peers in the following chapter.

CHAPTER 4

■ ■ ■

Enlisting Help from Parents, Teachers, and Peers

I know he's different, but he's also, like . . . just a boy, too.
—*CHRIS*, *age six*,
friend to David, who has autism

To have a playdate, or get invited to a birthday party, kids need to know and meet other kids. This may come naturally for typical children, but for children with autism, meeting other children is not an easy endeavor. Studies have shown that when given opportunities to interact, autistic children often choose to remain alone while typical children naturally move to join in and engage with each other socially. Children with autism, even those who seek solitude, do want to relate (albeit in their own way) with others. Unfortunately, their communication deficits and sensory processing difficulties get in the way.

Finding Friendship

Finding real friendship is difficult for autistic kids. Though most children do want to interact in their own time, many play situations and social exchanges with peers are forced, and it can be upsetting to parents to see their children give more undivided attention to objects and foods—rather than would-be friends and family members. Though the appearance of disinterest in interacting with others can be discouraging, I would rather you think of it as a temporary incapacity or shortcoming—not disinterest. The kids don't know what is available to them through friendship, what to do among others, or how to proceed appropriately with others, and many children with autism are hesitant to even experience the "feeling" of an interaction. This is why parents are important facilitators when it comes to encouraging their children to socialize more.

As you move with your child from school to therapy to the playground, you must tread carefully with your requests and examine your expectations of your child in social settings. Try to take notice of natural environments your child feels comfortable in (the pool, the library, the park, et cetera). Keep an eye out for possible buddies, and for other parents who welcome and are comfortable with diversity. Finding true friendship "possibilities" can be tricky. Unless your child is high functioning or has only mild spectrum-like qualities, his differences and quirks will be noticed. And typical children may ask you questions about your child that may give you uncomfortable twinges.

A peer who shows interest and curiosity in this way can still become a genuine friend for your child—so don't count out those who notice the autism.

Typical children are able to initiate friendships and playdates on their own, as they go about their daily activities at recreation centers, school playgrounds, and after-school sports. But it is harder for our autistic kids. A child with autism will, at least early on, need a parent, caregiver, teacher or therapist to be the initiator for him. If your child's social skills are not adequate enough to independently engage with a peer, or if your child is still young, your initiations for playdates will need to be addressed to the parents of the kids you would like your child to "formally" engage with. And this can be a little intimidating when you are unsure of what reactions you'll get from their parents.

Most of the time, things work out well. Reaching out to other parents can be rewarding and liberating not only to you, but also to the other parents. I have spoken with many parents of typical kids who have wanted to get to know or reconnect with the parents of special needs kids in their neighborhoods—as they want to invite the special needs children to their kids' parties and to their homes—but they are nervous about their own lack of knowledge and experience, and are afraid of either saying the wrong thing or keeping the special children safe. One mother of two typical elementary-aged children, when asked if she would feel comfortable inviting a child with autism over for a playdate, said, "I don't know if I would be able to take care of the child. To be honest, I feel like I would put my foot in my mouth around the kid's parents. I am so thankful my children are healthy and normal, but I wouldn't even be able to say that." Another mother of a typical elementary-aged daughter responded with, "I absolutely would feel fine about it. I am not the mother of a child with autism, but one day I may be a grandmother of a child with autism. Or an aunt of a child with autism." Parents of typical children have also mentioned that it is hard to get to know parents of special needs children (autism included) because their time is really spread thin with therapies and family responsibilities.

Finding friends for your child will involve answering those "wh" questions that those of us who live and work with children with autism know so well! The what, where, and who questions involved in finding playdates are not so easy to answer—but can be worked out in time.

One mother finds that her child's OT sessions offer the perfect opportunity not only for her son to be able to play with a peer, but for her to be able to have some adult contact and chats with other moms.

> I've invited other mothers and their kids to join me at the rehab center, which gives us a chance to talk while our kids play in a semistructured environment. It is my "let's meet for coffee" haven. It helps so much for me to be able to do it this way, because my time is limited, and my house is not clean most of the time. I am thankful the OT allows my son to have a friend at his sessions, and I am so thankful to now have a handful of mothers in my community that really do understand what I have to deal with—the good and the bad. Once they get to see and know my son, there is a level of comfort—where they just understand, and can relate to me as just another mother. I love that the other mothers get to see how much in common my son has with their own kids—even though their kids are typical.

Where to Start

You may be able to find potential playmates in the areas you frequent every day. The following are great places to begin:

- Your neighborhood street

- Your place of worship

- The local playground

- Your child's class at school

- Your local YMCA, YWCA, or recreation center

Keep your eye out for kids who are attracted to being with your child, and introduce yourself to the children's parents with the compliment of how friendly and helpful their kids are with your child. If they hadn't noticed, let them know your child has autism and struggles to make friends. Your compliment to their child and openness will almost always be positively received.

When looking for friendship possibilities in your child's class at school, ask the teacher for a class list with phone numbers and, if possible, one that includes the classmates' pictures. You should feel free to call others and introduce yourself, because students and their parents often use class lists to set up playdates. Ask your child if he can name someone from his class that he would like to play with, or choose a classmate you know. If there is a chance the classmate may feel confused by some of your child's behaviors, you may need to mention that your child's autism makes it difficult for him to socialize and approach other kids.

I know that a few of you may be cringing at my advice to bring up the autism and have such a conversation, but many parents of typical kids have mentioned that it is a relief when the parent of the child with autism talks about it. Both adults and children become very uncomfortable when it appears they are not supposed to mention a disability (or difference), or when they feel like they have to pretend or act like they don't see it. Of course, it is wonderful to highlight commonalities within the same conversation—both of our kids enjoy eating pizza, love animals, et cetera—and there is value, for the typical kids, in forming a friendship with your child. Typical kids often gain appreciation of their own abilities, as well as the hard work and perseverance their friend must endure. Even if your child has more severe autism, you may be surprised to know that it can mean the world to a typical kid to be someone your child will play with, smile at, or listen to. Typical kids do notice and rejoice in little victories.

Another option for playdates and friends is to seek out the special needs kids who attend your child's school or live in your community. Sometimes, children with special needs really connect with each other, share interests (especially when children are delayed and have less mature interests than their peers), and feel comfortable among one another because of the slower paces of language, movement, and requests. Though it is important for your child to have good role models to learn appropriate social nuances, true friends can have differences and different abilities.

Great kids are out there, and they can be good friends to your child.

Teachers and Therapists Can Help

Teachers and therapists are excellent resources for friendship possibilities because they work daily with a lot of kids and know which children may be "good bets" for playdates. They observe numerous children daily in school and therapeutic environments and know which kids mesh well with your child. They also often know the parents of the children and may be able to advise whether the family as a whole may be open to or available for social get-togethers.

Teachers and therapists are also excellent resources for activities your child and a peer can engage in together, and they can tell you important little pieces of information such as an estimated length of time your child may be able to remain engaged with others during play activities, and when and how to incorporate sensory breaks if needed. They may also be able to help you see where some additional prompting may be beneficial to help an activity run smoothly, and where you may need to run interference. For instance, if your child takes a common phrase literally ("I have butterflies in my stomach."), you may need to explain what the phrase means to avoid undue confusion.

Occupational therapists can help recommend sensory activities your child can engage in before, during, and after an activity, which can help your child to be at his or her best. Speech and language therapists, teachers, and psychologists can help recommend some typical social phrases to practice so that your child can communicate more comfortably during time with a friend.

How to Model for Typical Kids

Most parents would like their children with autism to reference their peers, and learn by watching their peers during social activities, but at first, when trying to establish new friendships, it is helpful for peers to be able to reference *you* as you engage with your child. Watching you speak with and guide your child gives them helpful information about how to communicate with him or her. Typical children watch carefully how adults speak with and handle children with differences. Your modeling will give them clues to the special prompting your child may need, or the subjects or areas best avoided. Your modeling will also give clues about your child's ability and able-ness. For instance, if you speak naturally with your child, the kids will, too. If you shorten your language, and gesture to your child, the kids will learn to do this, too.

The way your child follows your direction, and the way your child responds to you and plays, will be noted and used by your child's peers. These are the social cues that typical children pick up, and you must know that your mood and style with your child will be noticed. This opens up a wonderful learning opportunity for both you and the typical peers. After observing you with your child, a few encouraging words may be all it takes to open up the doorway for other children to stand in your place and relate to your child . . . and for your child to relate back. Ask the typical kids if they would like to meet your child, and whether they would like to join you in play. Ask the kids if *they* would like to see if they can get your child to join *them*. Give them helpful hints of advice with a smile—don't show your nerves if you are holding your breath.

Modeling is a useful tool for some behind-the-scenes work with your child, too. Your modeling how to play a game, take turns, kick a goal, or recite a Scout pledge can help your child see, understand, and then practice an expected skill, which will ultimately help him fit into and participate more in a social activity. We call this *previewing* an activity or *priming* for an activity. Some children that may not be able to perform a "whole" skill, but may be able to easily perform several parts or half of the skill. I will show you how to preview and break down tasks into doable pieces when we work with the I.D.E.A.L. process in Part Two.

Parents Supporting Parents

There is nothing like being able to lay it all on the line to other parents who have been there. And there are many parents who, through community autism organizations, school groups, or support groups, are willing to share their experiences so others do not have to reinvent the wheel. Parents who have children with autism or other special needs will listen to you, support you, and offer advice if you need it. No doubt your experiences will one day help another parent who is new to the world of parenting a child with autism.

Parents of typical children can be supportive of you, too, and your endeavor to find your child friends. They may not understand the race against time, the need to fill each day with activities and therapies that will bring about growth, and the anxiety about where your child will be two or ten years down the line . . . but most want to take part in some way—they just don't know how to help.

Parents of typical children have become much more aware of how often children are being afflicted with an autism spectrum disorder, and know that autism could appear in their own immediate and extended families. And most parents want their typical children to accept all kids—no matter if they have learning differences. Most parents would also like their children to take on helpful and empathetic roles in the lives of children who may need extra help.

By allowing your child to socialize among peers, and by inviting your child's peers to share in your world, you will be not only helping your own child to grow, but helping the playmates and typical role models to grow as well.

It is the same with other parents. Opening yourself up to receive help from other parents will benefit not only you, but them, too. It is important to give families the benefit of the doubt, set aside your hesitations and thoughts about reactions, and make that phone call, so that your child can begin to foster friendships with other kids. Here are some important tips:

- When you set up a playdate or an activity, you will want both your child and the other child to experience something they enjoy. You know your own child's preferred activities, but do you know what the other child likes? Is there an activity they could take part in that could include the preferences of both? Might they be able to swing, swim, eat, paint, play with animals, or play catch together? Do they both like to ride bikes or make cookies? You should feel comfortable making an extra phone call to find out some of these important details when planning for an enjoyable play experience.

- Once you have a scheduled date, it is important to invite the parent(s) into your home during the playdate or activity. You should not expect initially that parents will be comfortable dropping off their child to play with a child with autism. If you are going to another's house, do not expect to be able to simply drop off your child for a playdate. In the beginning, it will be helpful if you remain. As others get to know your child, they will understand how to communicate with your child and see beyond the autism. It is then that they may feel comfortable having her visit without your presence or let their child visit you without their supervision.

- Parents also support parents online. There are numerous websites devoted to autism issues, and many of the organizations that run these sights have seasonal or yearly events where families impacted by autism join together with a common cause and focus. Many families who have attended these events have met and remained in touch with other families, and continue to reconnect on their own. Many adult friendships have been made, and many a friendship has formed between the children. Not only have the children with autism participated in new friendships, but also their typical siblings have formed friendships with other siblings who understand their experiences better than most of their peers at home. Also, many online communities and discussion forums relating to autism or parenting offer support, advice, and opinions on a huge array of topics—including socialization.

• A challenge that parents face as their children start to socialize more with other kids and their families is handling the advice and questions that come up relating to discipline. Parents of children with autism are not usually able to discipline their children in ways that look the same or work the same as discipline techniques used with typical children. The ignoring of certain behaviors or sensory interventions can look questionable to many, and it is frustrating for the parents of autistic kids to have to try and explain their actions while trying to handle their kids in their times of need.

If you find yourself in this uncomfortable position, stick with your child's routines and sensory interventions. You can later mention that certain websites explain behavioral needs and techniques for children with autism, if other parents are interested in understanding more about what they just witnessed.

Involving Siblings

If you have children who are typical in your family, they will often have concerns about their brother or sister's well-being during social activities, and the trustworthiness of those who are engaging with their brother or sister. You may see them fluctuate between wanting to do activities independently of their autistic sibling, and wanting to be present at every activity their sibling takes part in to help guide and watch over them. Many typical siblings feel they need to be present and at their brother's or sister's side whenever a parent is not. Others may try to avoid any and every activity their siblings are involved in, because they feel embarrassed or ignored.

As you spend time planning social events and activities for your autistic child, you should involve siblings by asking for their ideas and input about activities. Siblings may like to be involved in the behind-the-scenes practice of social skills, as role models, in therapy, and during less formal practices with just the family. Ask—do not demand—if they would like to come along to an activity (if old enough to have a choice), and if they do not want to join you, ask what they may want to do instead during that time period. If they suggest something that is possible to do—let them do it. If a sibling feels like she is constantly forced to set aside her own wants and interests, resentment may result, and some acting out may ensue. If a sibling has some discomfort over not being present to watch over a brother or sister, open up a discussion about how new situations and new people can be uncomfortable for all of us at first—until new people get to know each other better. Tell her that it is important for children with autism, including her brother or sister, to meet new people and try new things—in fact, these are basic needs for everyone.

Enlisting Help from the Community

Your community or communities nearby may be great places to involve your child in social and recreational activities. Your local school system may have after-school enrichment activities your child could join independently if able, or join with the assistance of a paraprofessional or approved helper. Extended school year programs that offer camp-like sports or group activities can also help your child meet and get to know new friends. Local recreation centers, YMCAs, YWCAs, and places of worship may also have social groups or social opportunities for special kids already in place—some have formed groups specifically to meet the needs of children with autism.

Your child will be able to join in on most of the recreational activities your community or district has in place for all children. If you feel there is an activity or event your child may enjoy, call the recreational center, and let them know you would like to sign up your child with autism. (Some parents have told me that they don't like to divulge the autism diagnosis until the activity starts, for fear of being discriminated against, and closed out of the activity. I believe it is best to be honest. And there are laws to protect you and your child from questionable acts and circumstances.) Let them know you would like to work with them on the logistics of how to make the experience work successfully for all. Here are a few things you can do to start a good relationship with a community venue:

- Offer to speak with the leaders and instructors.

- Plan to bring some helpful (keep it simple, if possible) information on your child.

- Visit the venue where the activity will take place.

- Offer to be available by phone during the activity hours.

The center may ask you to attend or to arrange for a helper (either privately or through your school district) to attend with your child, so you may need to look at some time and money considerations when registering your child for an activity. Some children who qualify for special programs outside of their school districts may be able to get some assistance free of charge.

I often hear parents of autistic children describe how frustrating and fatiguing it can be to constantly have to take the helm, and educate those they and their children come across in their communities. Many speak of the dilemma of wanting to address the questions, looks, and unsolicited advice, while also wanting to ignore the inquiries and comments to remain focused on their child and family.

Be selective with your time and efforts. For those you feel may be perplexed or irritated by your child's behavior, it is a good idea simply to suggest a website that describes autism. Better yet, give them a business card with the URL of an autism website, and say nothing.

Once you are out in the community more, you will find numerous people who will be willing and happy to include your child and show him or her friendship. They just need to know who your child is, and how they can help. Make that phone call.

CHAPTER 5

▧ ▧ ▧

Pairing the Right Activities with the Right Reinforcements

He likes to run a lot. He runs after me and tries to tag me, and his mom gives him stickers if he tags me soft . . . If he does it [too hard], he doesn't get stickers. If he gets lots of stickers, he gets to have fish [crackers]. I tell him to tag soft, and I'll sit with him if he gets fish, because his mom gives me some, too.

—SAM, *age eight,*
friend to Lucas, who has PDD

When choosing social activities for kids with autism, we want to highlight their strengths and interests, so that they will be able to take part in and enjoy shared activities. It is also essential that there be "payoffs" for appropriate behaviors and good efforts, and that the children see these "payoffs" as desirable. The payoffs that I am speaking of here are the positive reinforcers we discussed in Chapter Three.

All of the information you have gathered to this point, we will begin to use here, as we look closely at which social and recreational activities may fit well with your child's individual personality and characteristics. I would like you to look back at your lists of preferred and nonpreferred activities, and your descriptions of your child's sensory sensitivities as we move forward and look at some common social and recreational activities, and choose reinforcers based on your child's unique needs.

Matching Strengths to Activities

You may be familiar with a little exercise from my first book, *A Parent's Guide to Developmental Delays*, where we look at a child's strengths and weaknesses to help us decipher what the child is good at, and what the child struggles with. I would like to do this exercise with you, because your child's strengths will help direct you toward activities he or she may truly enjoy. Your child's weaknesses can help you bypass certain activities, at least for the time being. All children, when they are able to use their strengths in recreation and in social situations, show more enjoyment and success within them.

So, take a piece of paper, and divide it or fold it in half. And at the top of one side write the word "Strengths" and at the top of the other side write the word "Weaknesses." Then ask yourself the following questions:

- What does my child do well?

- What does he or she enjoy doing every day? (Don't worry if it is stereotypical.)

- What do I enjoy about my child?

- What is happening when my child spontaneously joins others?

Now ask yourself these questions:

- What does my child avoid?

- What makes it difficult for my child to express him or herself?

- What behaviors confuse people?

- What embarrasses me when I'm out with my child?

The very personal and individual information you have just listed as part of this exercise will help you choose activities wisely. Different activities require different sets of skills, and the sensory environments of activities vary enormously.

Look over the following list while considering your child's strengths and weaknesses:

- *Low demand for social skills*: Ballet, bike riding, photography, swimming, going to the movies, painting, drawing, computer gaming, working with clay, gymnastics, rowing, knitting, pony riding, roller skating, jumping rope, and Frisbee throwing.

- *Low demand for understanding verbal directions*: Swimming, running, jogging, collecting, roller skating, jumping rope, and Frisbee throwing.

- *Structured and predictable*: Ballet, swimming class, martial arts class, yoga, and social groups for special needs children.

- *Rote and repetitive*: Craft making, woodworking, swimming, running, jogging, knitting, rowing, jumping rope, and Frisbee throwing.

- *Involves ordering*: Gardening, auto mechanics, and model kits.

- *Highly visual*: Painting, drawing, and computer gaming.

- *Highly sensory and auditory*: Learning to play an instrument and dancing.

- *Highly sensory and active*: Soccer, baseball, basketball, football, gymnastics, tennis, cooking, playing with animals, ice-skating, roller skating, jumping rope, and Frisbee throwing.

Now list three activity possibilities you think your child may enjoy:

1.

2.

3.

Look at your list of the three possibilities, and look back at the sensory information you had gathered in Chapter Two. Try to visualize what the sensory environments might be like within your activity choices. Do you need to possibly cross out one of your choices? Or are your choices well matched?

If you feel you have one or more activities your child could try, do the following:

- Find out if your choices are options in your community.

- Find out if there are same-age peers involved in the activities.

- Determine whether participation in one or more activities is financially feasible.

Recreational and leisure activities can be fun places for your child to practice his social skills, and once your child truly finds something he loves, he may stick with it and have a sport or hobby he carries with him through his youth, into adulthood.

How to Make an Activity Social

Within any activity, and within any setting, an activity is not social unless there is *reciprocity* between the participants. *Reciprocal interactions* can be challenging for children with autism because sustaining some sort of back-and-forth exchange requires several other skills including joint attention and visual or language processing. Reciprocal interactions may be verbal, as in a conversation, or may be action based, as in a game of catch. Many children, even when able to sustain some reciprocal interactions in the home, will need to be prompted or reminded of common phrases or rules in natural social environments. Often, kids will need to be prompted to attend to others, and prompted to respond to others' initiations.

Sustaining a reciprocal interaction is not, in and of itself, motivating to most children with autism. Many of the children will need the knowledge and motivating factor of an upcoming positive reinforcer to demonstrate reciprocal behavior—especially when activities or environments are new.

Priming for activities or prepracticing activities can help children take part in and demonstrate reciprocal interactions more readily. Modeling or role-playing sustained conversational interactions or play in your home can help your child develop an awareness of contributing and then responding; acting and then watching. You can prompt your child fully if needed, or at least partially, to help her successfully complete a simple interaction.

Language is often a hurdle for children with autism in social situations, so after you've primed your child, you may want to use pictures or written props as reminders. One way to do this is by writing *social scripts* for the child. Here is a simple example:

JAMES (written name or child's picture): Hi, Mrs. Smith.
MRS. SMITH (written name or person's picture): Hi, James, how are you?
JAMES (written name or child's picture): I'm fine.

This simple script may be written on a piece of paper or a large note card. James, the child with autism, would have his name near his lines, or if he didn't recognize his name, his picture would be placed near his lines (and you can also do this with the person the child is conversing with). His lines may also be highlighted with a highlighter, whereas the other person's anticipated lines would not be. For even more severe autism, social scripts can be modified with picture cues. One child I worked with a couple years ago was very quick to memorize social scripts and would use them independently only a couple of weeks after practicing them with the reminder cards. The confidence he felt from eliciting responses from others, after initiating a reciprocal interaction, became a powerful motivator for him.

I want to mention to you that when you become involved in activities and recreation in your communities where your child is a participant mostly among typical kids, it is easy to lose track of your social objectives for your child and the need for reciprocal interactions. The reason is that the skills of typical kids can be distracting, especially when your child's skills are not up to par. Parents and caregivers unintentionally begin to focus on getting their children to be able to perform as well as their peers, and often come away discouraged. This also doesn't help the children begin to forge new relationships, nor figure out where to fit in as a member of a whole.

When the focus within an activity is only on skill acquisition, children with autism are often taken aside for further instruction and guidance owing to the kids' communication issues. Though it is possible your child may end up being a star within her chosen activity, it is okay, too, to have your child take on an assistive or supportive role. For instance, in a cooking class, if a child is unable to work the range properly, or mix ingredients because of motor issues, she could hand the ingredients to a partner, or bring certain utensils to a partner when asked. These actions are reciprocal, and help children work together.

Using Preferred Objects and Reinforcements During Activities

Children's preferred objects, activities, well-loved books, TV shows, or movie characters can all be used in several ways to encourage successful participation in activities. One of the simplest ways to use preferred objects is to allow your child to bring one to an activity. If a preferred object is not age-appropriate, help your child find an alternative that can fit in a pocket or hook on to a belt loop. Sometimes wearing a sticker of a favorite character on one's hand or shirt does the (positive distraction) trick.

Preferred objects can also be used during transitions, if transitions are difficult. Here are a few ways to use them while transitioning:

- Read out loud to your child from his favorite book, and let him follow you as you move (transition) to a different area.

- Show your child a favorite toy, and let him know that he can hold the toy when he sits down "over there."

- Sing favorite songs or use active patterns while walking into unknown buildings or during transitions, which can help children with autism remain attentive (and remain with you), with satisfactory self-regulation.

Reinforcing your child's positive behavior, and the behaviors you want to keep, is vitally important. And we do this by using preferred objects as positive reinforcers. As we discuss these reinforcers in more detail, I would like you to either jot down or mentally take note of a few possibilities that may work for your own child.

As you reward your child for appropriate behaviors and/or responses, the rewards will either be *immediate* or *delayed*. Immediate rewards come the moment right after a wanted behavior occurs, while a delayed reward may come after earning five tokens, or after earning four puzzle pieces that together make up a picture of the reward. Positive reinforcements and rewards will also either be *connective* or *disconnective* when given during social activities.

Connective rewards do not disrupt a child's participation in an activity. The child does not leave the activity and does not have to move from the activity to receive the award. So, for instance, if we are rewarding a child by giving him a fish cracker, a hug, a high-five, or a token, the child can maintain his focus and participation within the activity, and hopefully continue on for a longer duration. These rewards may be called *embedded*.

Disconnective rewards do disrupt a child's participation in an activity, because they require movement to a different location, or a complete change in focus, to receive the positive reinforcer. When a child is expected to participate in an activity for only a small duration, he may then be rewarded with a break or a swing in a different room or location. These are examples of disconnective rewards.

It's important to make this distinction because a child who has difficulty transitioning may not be able to return to or rejoin a social activity after receiving a disconnective reward. Connective rewards work well as positive reinforcers during activities to increase the durations of good effort, cooperation, as well as good self-regulation and participation. Disconnective reinforcers are wonderful to use when children are showing effort, but their stamina is waning, or when the children can only regulate their bodies for a certain interval of time. Some parents use connective reinforcers for a span of time, and then use an ending disconnective reinforcer—to exit on a high note.

When choosing reinforcers for our children, we should have several ideas for both connective and disconnective rewards.

Let's look at some examples of connective rewards. Connective rewards can be either immediate or delayed. Here are some examples:

Spoken exclamations: *"Great job!"*
Edibles
High-fives
Hugs
Stickers
Tokens (most often for delayed reinforcements and
 rewards)
Points (most often for delayed reinforcements and
 rewards)
Puzzle pieces
Tickles
Smiley faces (hand drawn)
Checkmarks
Ink stamps

Here are some examples of disconnective rewards. Disconnective rewards are often delayed and earned over time. Examples include:

Going to the library
Going to the playground
Going to eat a snack in a separate location
Getting sensory input in a different location
Going through a restaurant drive-thru
Engaging in stereotopy in a different location
Being lifted or played with by a preferred person
Watching a DVD or TV program
Listening to music, separate from others

Listening to a book on tape, or listening while a
     preferred person reads
Going for a walk with a preferred person

Do you have a few reinforcements in mind that would work for your child? List them here.

Connective reinforcers:

1.

2.

Do you feel your child would initially need these as immediate reinforcers? Or would you be able to delay reinforcement and have her earn them with tokens or puzzle pieces?

Disconnective reinforcers:

1.

2.

Make sure the environment of your child's activity allows for your disconnective rewards.

Breaks and Escapes

When we take our kids into new environments, there are a lot of unknowns. And even when we entertain in our own homes or attend functions at the homes of family members, special events and activities can become overwhelming for our kids.

This is why we need to make sure that there are rooms or areas that we can designate as "quiet areas," "break areas," or "cool-down areas." When given the chance, a good number of our kids with autism can regain their composure after sensory discomforts, tantrums, and outbursts, if given the chance to regroup and rest. Some children feel the need to hide away in the midst of sensory input and the unique "feels" of environments—feelings we may not be aware of. When attending activities or events, children should be primed and told where the quiet area or break area will be. You can work out a verbal or nonverbal (sign or picture) system with your child, so she can tell or show you when she needs a break. You can let your child know that if she has an outburst, there is a room she will go to until the outburst is over.

It has been helpful for some parents to actually arrive a little early to an activity or event, and to go to the designated "quiet area" to sit or have a snack. This can help children with autism become a little more acclimated to the surroundings, and can help the children have a smoother transition into the special activity—and possibly avoid the commotion of the arrival of others.

Check out the locations of recreational activities beforehand and work out a space for a quiet area or break area with recreational staff, if you feel your child may need it. A quiet area can be a large tree near the soccer field, so there is some flexibility when venues are short on space.

Remain Alert for Changes in Preferred Activities

One day, you may notice that the Pokémon stickers don't seem to be doing the trick anymore, and that your child is pushing the envelope and acting inappropriately. It is important to remain alert to when reinforcers are just not as "reinforcing" as they used to be. The truth is our children grow, new movies come out, and new books are read, and suddenly the obsessions that brought good behavior and lots of stars on the activity charts have shifted to other obsessions. Monthly, you should reevaluate your child's preferred activities and favorite media characters, because you want to be able to use them to keep your child's motivation high.

As your child grows, his nonpreferred activities may change as well. The terror when in proximity of the swimming pool may turn into a much less harrowing cautious curiosity, which we can work with.

The next part of this book will be about taking action. I hope you will jump right in as we begin to learn the I.D.E.A.L. process for being socially included.

Previewing

and Planning Using

I.D.E.A.L. Elements

TWO

CHAPTER 6

■　　■　　■

I.D.E.A.L.

I: Introduce an Activity

When we go somewhere, we have to tell him what it is and what happens there before we go, or he freaks out. We can't just bring him. It's kind of like he's activity blind.

—*SETH*, *age eight,*
big brother of James, who has autism

It is time to take action. And armed with your knowledge of your child's unique sensitivities, and strategies for handling difficult situations and behaviors, you are now ready to begin using the I.D.E.A.L. system, which will help you prepare for and carry out social plans and activities with your child. By giving some consideration to and taking action on each of the five different steps that make up I.D.E.A.L., you will optimize the possibility your child will be able to successfully engage in social activities and events.

I.D.E.A.L. is an acronym, and each letter stands for a different, yet equally vital, preparation step, which together can prepare your child with autism to enter into and participate in natural social environments.

I: stands for Introduce the Activity
D: stands for Determine the Tasks Involved
E: stands for Evaluate Your Expectations
A: stands for Accommodate for Success
L: stands for List the Activity Components Visually

When all five tasks are completed, you will find that you will be able to more successfully include your child in social situations, as well as anticipate the possible problems that may arise—even if your child has very little social experience.

In this first step in the I.D.E.A.L. process, you will learn to (**I**) introduce activities to your child *before* he takes part in them. We will devote the entire chapter to learning how to complete this step in a way that works for your individual child.

We want to introduce activities *prior* to your child's participation, because it is very comforting for a child with autism to know what is going to happen *beforehand*. I cannot emphasize enough the importance of this first step. Many, many negative behaviors arise in children with autism solely because the kids do not know what to expect, or do not understand what is happening—or happening around them. Some autistic children, in their confusion, anticipate the possibility of sensory pain or discomfort. Communication difficulties, elements of surprise, noises, demands, and discomforts can all provoke severe reactions that can make socializing almost impossible. This is why the simple step of previewing and priming for what is to come is so beneficial. Previewing and priming your child for upcoming activities will increase his or her ability to self-regulate, cope, and understand what is expected.

Previewing Is Crucial

One of the hallmarks of children who have any ASD is an inflexibility in their ability to adapt to varied types of change or demands. It is also difficult for children with autism to shift their focus. It can be simply overwhelming for many of the children to be led into unknown environments or to have new demands placed on them—especially when already stressed. Children with autism need time to slowly process and prepare themselves for different experiences, and time with different people. They need time to adjust, and they need tools to help them understand what will be happening before demands are made to perform in some way.

Children with autism have unique skills that are individual from one another, so I will be introducing several techniques to preview activities. These different options have varying requirements for language processing, and some options are highly visual in nature. With a little experimentation, I believe you will find one that will work well for your child.

Visits and Photographic Walks

One way to preview an activity with your child or prime her for an outing is to visit the location of the activity or event on a day prior to its scheduled date. Bringing your child with you on the visit is beneficial, unless it is *your* first visit to the venue or house, and you are not sure what to expect. You should bring or borrow a camera, and take pictures of the actual places, environments, people, and materials your child will see upon her participation. If your child is with you, you can take pictures of her in the different environments, and among some of the different people she will be with.

Next print out your pictures, and make a little book using note cards or construction paper. At a quiet time, when your child is able to attend, flip through the pictures or book together, and talk about each picture and what she will be expected to do in each location and with each person. This is called taking a photographic walk. If you can get a staff member or family member to tell you beforehand what the order of events will be, place the pictures on a strip of cardboard or in a hand-made book in sequential order. This will allow for an even better, more concrete understanding of what's to come.

Using and Writing "Social Stories"

"Social stories" are short, matter-of-fact narratives that help children with autism comfortably preview or learn about upcoming activities and common situations. The use of the phrase "social structures" will be used in this book to represent short priming stories for introductory and transitional uses. Because the stories are simple and reassuring, your child can be introduced to and prepared for new situations that may cause anxiety or confusion.

You can write your own "social stories" that describe what will happen during a future activity, in the form of a short personal narrative. It is important that you use words and language your child is familiar with and understands. If your child has difficulty processing spoken language, he will also have difficulty processing "social stories."

One way to help kids whose language processing is low is to incorporate pictures and photos into the story. Using "social stories" on a regular basis can help to facilitate language growth. You can combine a "social story" with your photographic walk.

"Social stories" are very versatile—not only can you use them to introduce a new situation, but you can also be creative, teaching your child expected behaviors while describing the future event. For instance, you can write a "social story" for an upcoming playdate, and include the verbal greeting you would like your child to say as part of the story.

Here are examples of "social stories" written for two different language processing levels. Both will introduce the same activity—a playdate with a friend.

LOWER LANGUAGE

Steven is coming to **play**. **He** is my **friend**. **I** will **show Steven animals** and **cars**. **It is okay** if **Steven touches** my **animals** and **cars**. **First, I** will **play animals** and **cars** with **Steven**. **Then, I** will **eat cheese puffs** with **Steven**. **Then, Steven** will **go home**.

The key words in bold, which were familiar to the autistic child in the story, were used to foster understanding.

The following "social story" could be used with a child who has more advanced language skills.

HIGHER LANGUAGE

My friend, Steven, is coming to my house today. He is coming at one o'clock. I will say, "Hi, Steven," when he comes. I will show Steven my toys, like my animals and cars. Steven might want to play with the computer or play outside, and that's okay. Then I can make a choice and play with Steven or play by myself for ten minutes. Next, Steven and I will have cheese puffs for snack. Then it will be time for Steven to go home. I will say, "Thanks for coming, Steven!"

Some like to take the "social story" and break it up into parts that the child can check off as he performs each part.

Using and Writing Bubble Books

Bubble books also introduce new situations and can be used to preview activities. The word "bubble" comes from the circles around the verbalizations and thoughts that we see in comics. Bubble books, themselves, are written in the form of a comic, with visual characters (which are sometimes stick figures) who speak, think, and demonstrate tasks. Some children with autism really love this form of introduction, but it does not work well for all. The children must be able to follow a visual sequence (some will be able to do this with a little help) and process the language. The visuals in bubble books help children understand the language used.

Like picture books where you take photographic walks, bubble books, in their comic strip form, break activities or lessons into a sequence of steps. Bubble books do not need to be professionally made or written and drawn by only talented artists. Kids love the stick figures parents draw into the comics, too.

Role Playing and Video Modeling

Both role playing and video modeling are used to help teach children new social skills, but they are also great introductory and previewing tools. You can role-play in the privacy of your own home the difficult situations that may come up in new activities, as well as discuss problem-solving solutions and appropriate language.

Video modeling is a powerful tool, for you can videotape different environments and the people in them, giving kids a real-life feel for where they are headed. Children can become familiar with not only the visual aspects of the environments and people, but also with the sounds and the auditory aspects of the noise levels and voices they will need to attend to. When children with autism are videotaped (or digitally recorded) within social situations, and can later watch themselves (repeatedly, if needed) interacting among others, some really do notice and can label when they are acting appropriately and inappropriately. Some children with autism will purposefully try to adjust their behavior after viewing themselves on videotape. All of us would, if we watched ourselves on videotape, want to possibly adjust our behaviors in certain situations or when among certain people.

You can bring in the role playing as a generalization tool after a child sees himself on videotape or watches an activity he will soon be attending. Siblings often enjoy getting involved in the role playing of appropriate behaviors and the filming of different locations.

When There Are Unexpected Changes in Plans

Parents dread last-minute changes, especially when their kids are particularly rigid and have transitional meltdowns. But the reality is, things happen: thunderstorms come, playmates come down with strep, and fender benders happen on the way to the pool. When unforeseen circumstances come up, and unexpected changes in plans happen, it is important to be prepared. This may mean having some preferred items with you, such as toys, favorite foods, or a portable DVD player with a favorite movie. No matter where you are when the unexpected occurs, it is beneficial to write a new "social story" or bubble book "on the fly" to simply and clearly explain the changes to your child.

Here is an example of a quick "social story" to explain a change in plans:

> Steven was coming to my house to play. He is sick. He is in bed at his house. Sometimes kids get sick and have to stay home. Steven wants to come play at my house when he is better. His mom will take care of him and tell us when he is better.

In a situation like this, after the "social story" is read, give your child a choice of possible activities, so he or she will know how to proceed and know what to do next.

It is also helpful to carry a write-on wipe-off board with you at all times you are away from your home, because you can use it for whatever visual need comes up—whether it be a "social story," activity list, bubble book, or emergency behavior chart—and you can make and use it quickly with your child. You do not need a large board—one the size of a standard sheet of paper or one that is half that size and fits in your handbag should work fine.

Action Step for the **I** in **I.D.E.A.L.**

Did you feel a certain type of introduction would work well for your child? To help you decide, check off which of the following pertains to your individual child's needs:

VISUAL

_____ Sequenced and Ordered Visuals Needed
_____ Some Visuals of the Environment Needed
_____ A Visual for Attending Purposes Only Needed

LANGUAGE

_____ Understands Only Simple and Familiar Words
and Phrases
_____ Understands Most Literal Sentences
_____ Understands Natural Language

For children with lower language levels, you can choose highly visual modes of introduction, such as photographic walks and video introductions. Kids with higher and more natural language may find a lot of comfort and enjoyment in "social stories" and role playing.

When you have introduced and previewed an activity with your child, you have completed the first step in the I.D.E.A.L. process.

CHAPTER 7

▦ ▦ ▦

I.D.E.A.L.

D: Determine the Tasks Involved

I tell her to do just one thing at a time, and if she doesn't know how, I help her.

—KATE, *age nine*,
friend of Ashley, who has PDD–NOS

We may not realize it readily, but a small task that seems very simple to you and me may feel like a frustrating maze of complex steps for children with autism. Even the simple act of greeting "the birthday boy" at a birthday party involves a series of steps that must be followed precisely in order to make the interaction successful. For example, first, the child must spot and recognize the correct friend. Next, the child must self-regulate him or herself while moving across a room or yard to that friend, without being distracted or flustered by noises and movement. After that, the child must get the friend's attention, either vocally or by initiating a gentle touch (exerting the right pressure—making sure it does not feel like a push). Lastly, the child has to make eye contact and have something to say—such as "Happy Birthday!"—with an appropriate voice inflection and facial expression.

We will learn in this chapter how to take a larger task and break it into lists of sequential steps or *little* tasks. This will help you determine steps within a task your child will be able to perform independently, and steps you will have to prompt or assist. By analyzing tasks in this way, you will gain a clear picture of where your child will be successful (and not successful). This will, in turn, help you to set realistic expectations for your child as he enters into social situations.

Analyzing Tasks

All tasks, from washing one's hands, to setting the table, to cooking a meal, to making a foul shot, can be broken into small pieces or components that, when listed in order, make up a whole, complete task. If you watch yourself as you perform your own tasks throughout the day, and really pay attention to the different parts or details of what you are doing, you will see that making a phone call, getting the mail, and showering require many different motor tasks, judgments, and possibly communication skills that may be less automatic and really difficult for your child to do.

Analyzing a task is the basis for forming a *task analysis*, where you list each step in an activity or task, and know that your finished product will yield the completion of the activity or task. If you look at each step you have listed, and follow them yourself to see if you indeed reach your objective, which is the completion of the task, you will see that you have a chain or string of different "little steps" that make up what most of us see as "one" task.

Task analysis is extremely useful for children with autism, because, although the kids may not be able to handle an entire task on their own, they most certainly may be able to handle one or more of the smaller components of the task. And as the kids grow in their experience and familiarity with a task, more of the pieces or components can be added to their repertoires. The remaining components may need to be prompted or assisted.

The information on what pieces children can perform independently is vital because children with autism, when joining activities and social events, may be able to perform parts of tasks they cannot completely handle on their own. This way, expectations for the child can be clear, and someone can jump in to assist at certain times if needed. Task analysis can help autistic children learn new skills and establish greater independence.

Here is an example of a task analysis for brushing one's teeth:

Take red toothbrush.
Turn on cold water.
Put white brush part in water.
Count to 3.
Turn off water.
Take toothpaste.
Take cap off toothpaste.
Squeeze toothpaste out onto white brush part.
Brush toothpaste all over teeth in mouth.
Count to 25 in mind's voice.
Spit out toothpaste.
Turn on water and fill cup.
Put water in mouth and swish.
Spit out water.

Wash toothbrush in water.
Put toothbrush away.
Put cap on toothpaste.
Put toothpaste away.

This simple task was broken down into many components, and I want to impress upon you that some kids need their tasks broken into tiny components, as above. A child with autism may or may not understand what "brush your teeth" entails or even the steps that it takes to "rinse." By writing out *all* the components of the activity or task you want your child to perform, you will be able to check off the pieces he or she is able to complete on his or her own. For instance, your child may be able to do the first seven steps on her own, but falter when it comes to the acts of brushing and rinsing. You can then look at your list and see clearly which steps your child will need to be taught. Simple things we do daily are not always so simple for children with autism.

Some children use the chaining of steps in a task analysis as reminders for sequence and order. They may only require an abbreviated version of the same task:

Take toothbrush.
Wet toothbrush in water.
Put toothpaste on toothbrush.
Brush teeth.
Rinse mouth.
Rinse toothbrush.
Put things away.

For children who are unable to read or recognize the steps on a task list, we can pair words with visuals, or create visuals that depict each of the components.

Let's look at a different example—one involving an activity. When we analyze tasks for social or recreational activities, our task analysis may look something like this one, which depicts checking out books from the library:

Look at books.
Choose two books.
Tell adult "Ready."
Walk with adult to checkout desk.
Wait for turn.
Give worker library card and books.
Wait for worker.
Take library card and books.
Walk with adult to waiting place.

Again, as parents analyze the task, they may find that their child can complete several steps of the task independently, but not all. A child may be able to look for books, and choose books completely independently, but he may need assistance locating the checkout desk and handing over his chosen books momentarily. Some children may need support for the steps that require "waiting," such as understanding that one must wait in line for one's turn, or that others may not be finished choosing *their* books.

Independent and Supported Steps

As we break different tasks into smaller components and take a close look at the many steps even small tasks require, we will often see that the kids will be able to perform certain components independently and certain components only with our help. It is

#70   02-23-2013 2:01PM
Item(s) checked out to p14379430.

TITLE: The socially included child : a p
BARCODE: 3 1379 02164 7749
DUE DATE: 03-16-13

Tredyffrin Public Library

okay for your child not to have a task's or activity's entire sequence of skills down. If you allow your child to do what she can do independently and assist with the steps your child needs to learn, you will see a familiarity grow with those codependent parts. And with familiarity, you may see your child begin to exert more independence. It is important to keep track of which components your child is able to do independently, and which components still require help. The goal is to *eventually* get your child to be able to perform each component so that she will be able to perform the entire task or activity independently. Please, though, do not think that simply writing a task analysis will bring about independence—it requires modeling and work to master each small step in a greater task.

Assisting with Prompting

The help that we give kids when they falter with skills or when they need assistance to complete steps within a task is called a *prompt.* A prompt is simply a mini-intervention that helps a child to perform or do something he is unable to perform or do on his own. Prompts may be:

- Verbal

- Gestural

- Physical

- A combination of the above

Prompts may also be *full* on, where, for instance, a child may need full and complete physical guidance through a task step, or only *partial*, where, for instance, a child may just need the first sound of a friend's name (the sound "b" for the name "Bobby") given to remind him to say "Bobby." You may hear professionals say, "I needed to give him full physical prompting for the first step, but only partial verbal prompting for the next one."

It is very common for parents to find that a combination of prompts work well, as in the use of verbal prompts with gestures. Gestures help by allowing kids' to use their visual abilities to help them process information.

Once we are prompting the children through the more difficult parts of the tasks, we need to plan ahead for how we will eventually eliminate the prompts, because the kids will (happily) become reliant on our involvement and helpfulness if we continue to take charge with what is most difficult for them.

Fading Prompts

When we want our children to learn to be independent with areas we are prompting, we begin to fade the prompts we are giving. This is called *prompt fading.* Although there may not be an exact moment when you will know that your prompting can be faded, it is beneficial to gradually reduce the prompting a little bit at a time. By going through the process of pulling back on your assistance a little, or going from full to partial prompts, *you will learn to know* how close your child is to independence.

If you are verbally or physically prompting your child, you can plan to slowly decrease your speech and language cues to simple sounds, or decrease your physical prompts from full hand-over-hand help to a touch on the hand. If you are using a combination of prompts, such as verbal prompts with gestures, switch to gesture only, and gradually decrease from there.

If your child is unable to perform the task step with the faded prompts, you may need to practice the skill with the full on prompts longer.

Generalization of Isolated Skills

You may have analyzed the tasks of toileting and hand washing and worked with your child until she performed most of the steps independently in your house, but upon entering a recreation facility's bathroom or your friend's bathroom, the change in environment and the different-looking toilets seem to throw your child off. If this happens, don't be surprised. Skills that are learned in isolated environments can be difficult to generalize. Most children with autism need additional practice in new environments to perform skills that they readily perform in familiar places (and with familiar people) like home.

It is helpful to use the same task list, and the prompting your child is accustomed to, so that your child can learn that a task can be performed in the same way in many different locations. Sometimes using a "social story" works well in letting children know that toilets may look different in different places, but we use them in the same ways—just like the one he is accustomed to at home.

Action Step for the **D** in I.**D**.E.A.L.

I would like you to choose an activity or task that you feel would be beneficial for your child to be able to do independently. Then take the activity or task and *analyze* it. Maybe this would be greeting another, passing out a snack, helping to make cookies, or joining in on play. Write down the name of the task, and then list each sequential step that your child would need to accomplish to successfully complete the task. You can use the space provided, or do this on a separate piece of paper. This is just practice, so give it a try!

Task: _____

   1.

   2.

   3.

   4.

   5.

   6.

   7.

   8.

   9.

10.

Follow the steps you've come up with in order, and see if you complete the task! The more you practice analyzing tasks, the more you will begin to automatically see tasks as a sequence of doable parts—which make up a whole. This will no doubt benefit your child.

One you have taken an activity and have determined the sequence of tasks involved, you have completed the second step in the I.D.E.A.L. process.

CHAPTER 8

■　■　■

I.D.E.A.L.

E: Evaluate Your Expectations

My mom gets mad when Brandon starts flapping and won't talk
or look at anyone because he isn't out of control like that at
home. Sometimes when we go out, he gets really scared or acts
different. I don't know if he does it because he doesn't want to
be out. I don't know why he does it.

—*CHARLIE*, *age eight,*
little brother of Brandon, who has autism

It is common for children with autism to experience extreme
anxiety in social situations, and the discomforts they feel make
it hard for them to perform skills they've already mastered and
practiced in nonsocial or therapeutic environments. Therefore,
setting realistic expectations for autistic children in social settings
can be challenging.

New environments and new demands do impact skill use

and performance. For example, dealing with the environmental stimuli while trying to cognitively put together a sequence of words that make sense can fatigue an autistic child quickly. The internal multitasking kids with autism have to do in social settings can result in the deterioration of their moods as well as their desire to take part at all.

Look at Durations

Every activity or event takes place within a span of time—maybe one hour, maybe three hours—and to help children with autism successfully take part, we need to find out these time periods beforehand, as well as what will be happening. This will allow for you to make sound judgments about how much time your child may be able to handle, or how you may need to break up the time with snacks, rests, or sensory breaks.

I really want you to understand that the duration of an activity, by itself, can affect the success of a child with autism. Sometimes autistic kids will do well for a period of time, but run into trouble down the road as they tire, begin to feel hungry, or overtax their sensory systems. When you plan ahead, you can avoid this.

Children do not need to participate for the full time period of an activity or event. Perhaps, they could attend for the first half hour, or attend during the last hour. It is better to go for a successful small chunk than a larger span that may be overwhelming.

If you look back at the information you collected on your child's daily moods, you may see a time period where your child is at his best that matches up to the time of a recreational activity your child may enjoy. Use your observations of durations of "on" behavior in your house to help estimate durations that could be spent out. If your family is invited to a dinner or to a party, possibly attend for the hour your child is more "available" and interactive. If you (**I**) introduce the activity, and (**D**) determine the tasks involved, you may be able to smoothly make it through a short duration, and this could make for a positive experience that will build not only your child's confidence, but yours as well.

If you are unsure of the time durations your child may be able to handle, start with a relatively short period, because you want to optimize your child's possibility for success in the social situation. See how she does, and from even one outing, you will gain helpful information on how long your child can keep it together in subsequent social outings.

You will probably see your child's durations of participation in social activities begin to extend and grow over time. With repeated exposure, a growing feeling of familiarity will be fostered—with the environment, its characteristics, and the people who are present.

Your Emotions Play a Role

Though children with autism have well-known difficulties in labeling and noticing certain emotions, many autistic kids can be quite keyed into the moods and emotions of those who are important to them. As you introduce new ideas and activities to your child, and as you venture out socially, *your* mood may have an effect on the success of an activity. Kids pick up on a lot, and even though many may carry a diagnosis of autism, they are still kids. If you are anxious about bringing your child to an activity or playdate, or nervous about an upcoming event at your own home, you may be passing on a feeling of tension, which can and will be felt by your child. The kids may not be able to understand or define it—but even kids who are severely disabled will feel it.

Upon arriving at a new activity, if you are anxious about handing your child over to a staff member, your child may "get the message" and become noncompliant and oppositional, or he may tantrum or bolt. Basically if your child feels like you are not sure about the person, he will not want to go with that person. If you act irate toward a person he is supposed to go with, your child will not want to go with that person. The best moods for transitioning over to new people are matter-of-fact moods, friendly moods, and encouraging moods. If you need to do a little acting, do it.

None of this is easy at first. And kids with autism are at many different skill levels, so it really is less stressful for some than others. But the anxiousness about entering your child into new situations and the fear of them meeting failure in some way is the same.

You may not have had time to even take a moment to stop and think about your feelings about getting your child out there meeting new people and trying new things, but it is important to take a minute and remind yourself of all the why's—the reasons that propel you to want to do this for your child. Any new steps you take, as a result of new knowledge, *will* help your child, and I have great respect for your efforts and your dreams.

As you take your child out and encourage him to join in, with meltdowns or no meltdowns, remind yourself of your reasons (even write them down and put them away so that you can look at them whenever you need a little boost), and understand that there are no failures. Something may work well, and something else may not. Use the phrase "I will take note of this," and adjust if you have to for a more successful second or third outing. There should be no embarrassment or guilt in your preparations and phone calls to staff, family, or friends. There is just time to learn, grow, love your kids and family, and do the best that you can.

So when the anxious feelings crop up, take a minute in a quiet place and really look at them. Review those reasons that are personal to you—for doing what you are doing, and then go give your child a big hug.

Goals of Participation and Engagement

When you are involving and encouraging your child in social situations and activities, keep your eyes on the interacting. You want your child to grow socially, so you are aiming for participation, reciprocal interactions, and joint attention. This is not the time to bring in all of your child's IEP objectives, and the therapeutic expectations of using a correct pencil grip, using five-word utterances as opposed to two or three, or holding eye contact for certain amounts of time. (You will notice, however, that many of the skills your child works on in those educational environments will ultimately benefit your child if the skills are generalized.) It is important to be exposed to peers in social situations and to be able to self-regulate and be around others even before all of the discrete skills are generalized. Don't wait.

Before entering into an activity or event, think carefully about what you really want your child to accomplish. Then decide if it is a realistic expectation for your child. Has your child done it before? Then think about what you can do to help make it possible. Write a task analysis and really look at which steps your child can do independently, and which steps will have to be assisted.

For some parents, just having their child remain at the table during a special family dinner would feel like a major accomplishment. Others may see going to a local playground without their child launching into a tirade of screaming as a major success. One mom said that if her child would just greet his grandparents when they arrive for a visit, this would be success.

Look at your expectations, and look at your child's skills in your home. Your child will probably *not* use all of her skills when in new situations or among less familiar people. But *your child has the ability to*. It will just take a little time.

Tools for Targets

Once you have decided how you would like to see your child participate within an activity, and have carefully considered your expectations for independence and behavior, you can gather together your bag of tricks to help your child through rough spots and to prompt your child during steps that need assistance.

For instance, a trip with a friend to the pool that usually ends with your child having a tantrum upon leaving the water may need a few adjustments. Let's suppose one of your expectations is to leave the pool with the others, without having to bodily carry out your screaming child. (That would feel like success!) You would first (**I**) introduce the activity to your child with an emphasis on the expected exit behavior. Maybe this would be a photographic walk depicting in one picture a child exiting quietly (and then receiving a reward). Maybe using a "social story" would work well for your child. Then, you would (**D**) determine the tasks involved. Let's take a look at this:

TASK: LEAVING THE POOL

Get out of the water.
Walk and get dry towel.
Put on flip-flops.

Walk with Mom and friend into the locker room.
Walk with Mom and friend to car.

Here's where I need you to pay close attention. We now need to (**E**) evaluate our expectations. The expectation of your child doing this quietly when the habitual behavior is screaming may or may not be realistic. We need to look at the screaming. When does it occur? Where exactly is it occurring? Is there an obvious reason for the screaming? There are many possibilities, and here are a few:

- Your child is screaming because he wants to stay in the water and not get out.

- Your child is screaming because upon immediately getting out of the water, he can't stand the feel of his bathing suit sticking to his skin and legs.

- Your child is screaming because immediately upon leaving the water, he feels like he has to urinate.

- Your child is screaming because he has trouble walking barefoot on the warm or slippery pool deck.

- Your child is screaming because he cannot stand the anticipation of the feel of flip-flops on his wet feet.

As you can see, the true reason for the screaming could be solved as long as we pay close attention to why it is happening. We can help optimize our kids' chances for success by paying close attention in this way. If your child is verbal, perhaps your child can tell you at a later, quieter moment why he was so upset. But don't be surprised if he is unable to tell you (even if he is verbal). Answering "why" questions or questions involving personal feelings can be very difficult for children with autism. Let's look at some of the solutions you can use to help with this situation:

- Bring a timer and set it to go off when it is time to get out. As the timer rings, show your child a visual of an immediate reward (which must be preferred by your child, so you'll know he'll want it) he will get upon getting his towel.

- Have a helper hold a towel as a visual blocker, and have a dry bathing suit at your side as you do a quick lift and change, where your child's bathing suit will be removed upon being lifted out. Immediately put the dry bathing suit on and leave the area.

- Show your child a visual first-then board, depicting that first he will urinate and then he will receive a reward. Have your child urinate immediately before entering the pool, and give him a reward. When it is time to go, show him the board again, and quickly bring him to where he can urinate and then, again, give him a reward.

- You can keep a separate pair of dry pool shoes to put on, or upon getting out of the pool, immediately dry your child's feet and put on his everyday shoes. Or give him a piggyback ride to dryer ground.

As you can see, there are also many possibilities for solutions that may help bring about a more successful exit.

It is very common to overlook aspects of activities that are not goal oriented. Sometimes it is the rest times and the transition times that we have to plan for more. Many children with autism have great difficulty during the times that are less structured. A child with autism may begin pushing or punching during "free play," or may bolt suddenly instead of waiting for the door to be opened on the side of the car. These "lull" moments need to be planned for. Possibly, a staff member could take the lead during free play and start a group game. To lessen the chance of bolting during a "lull," the child could be given a special job—such as carrying something heavy to the car. He can then be positively reinforced for the helpful behavior.

Your observations together with your efforts to organize what you know, and what you know you will need, will, in every situation, benefit your child. The best tool to reach your targeted expectations is your preplanning.

Action Step for the **E** in I.D.**E**.A.L.

List two social situations or activities your child participated in—and did well:

1.

2.

Write on the lines below what you believe contributed to your child's success:

_____

_____

List two social situations or activities your child participated in—and did not do well:

1.

2.

Write on the following lines the details that made your child's experience unsuccessful:

_____

_____

Now that it is after the fact, can you think of some creative strategies you could have used to avoid those details that hindered your child's success?

_____

_____

Were your expectations realistic for your child?

_____

_____

I hope this excrcise has given you some useful information. We will learn more about the strategies that can help your child succeed in the next chapter.

By carefully evaluating your expectations for your child as related to certain activities, you have completed the third step in the I.D.E.A.L. process.

CHAPTER 9

■ ■ ■

I.D.E.**A**.L.

A: Accommodate for Success

He has his own iPod that he always carries with him, and if
there's too much noise somewhere, he'll put on his earphones
and listen to his favorite music. I wish my mom would get me my
own iPod.

—*GRANT, age ten,*
friend of Nathaniel, who has Asperger's syndrome

Accommodating activities for success involves manipulating
environments and shaping tasks so that children have a
greater chance of succeeding in them. Through accommodations, children with autism may be able to relate better, tolerate
an activity longer, and participate more.

In this chapter, I will explain to you how to make accommodations. You can use your task analyses and proposed expectations
for an activity to determine where changes must be made, or

where allowances need to be put into place to support your child's success.

An accommodation may be as simple as having a "quiet birthday table" where children sing "Happy Birthday" in their "whisper voices," so that the child with autism feels comfortable participating, too. An accommodation may be asking the lifeguard to warn you in advance before blowing the whistle to announce that free swim is over. This would allow you and your child to leave the pool area prior to the uncomfortable sound. An accommodation may be bringing a special lightweight ball to a bowling party, or bringing noise-canceling headphones to a soccer match. Perhaps you may only need to prepare and bring different foods for your child who is on a special diet.

We can accommodate children with autism in many different ways. Making accommodations can set kids up for success because it forces us to look at details such as the length of an activity, the number of people who will be there, the location of the activity, the food served, and the types of games to be played. By considering the **A** in I.D.E.**A**.L., your brainstorming will lead to solutions for accommodating possible trouble spots that might upset your child's ability to participate. I am excited that after reading this chapter, you will know how to make some accommodations that will make your child's social experiences more comfortable and positive.

Accommodation versus Assimilation

An *accommodation*, by definition, is "something supplied for convenience or to satisfy a need." During activities and social situations, we want children with autism to have many of these "somethings," so that their needs can be met. If a child can be helped by giving her accommodations, so that she does not have to put all of her concentrated efforts and focus on simply holding it together, she will be more available for interacting and attending to those in the environment. Accommodating kids in social environments helps them to navigate their experiences more successfully.

In contrast, *assimilation* is "to be taken into a larger whole and made similar." We can liken assimilation to being welcomed into a culture, or being absorbed into a group and made to belong. Of course, we want our kids to be respected for their individualities, and their ideas that are unique to each of them, but many understand the wish for children with autism to be able to assimilate with their same-age peers, and assimilate later in their lives, among adult friends, and among those in the workforce. Assimilation is a goal we can work toward with the kids, but accommodations are concrete things we can do right now. Possibly, as you get out more and give your child more experience in social settings, some of your kids will begin to assimilate more quickly than expected. But for some of us, it will be a long road, and though we would like to climb into the DNA of our kids and turn on those genes that may be dormant, we will have to exercise patience, and show the kids how very joyful being with others can be.

Strategic Placing of Accommodations

The way we decide what accommodations to use with the kids—basically where to supply those "somethings" that will satisfy their needs—is by, first, looking at the possible trouble spots in the upcoming activities and environments. Trouble spots are often due to:

• Sensory issues

• Communicative issues

• Cognitive and comprehension issues

• Stamina and fatigue issues

• Physical and motor issues

• Food allergy and sensitivity issues

Though the thought of accommodating your child or asking for accommodations may seem a little overwhelming, many accommodations are simple, logical, and easy to do. Once parents start using accommodations for trouble spots, they find that outings and social activities run more smoothly for everyone involved.

There are two types of accommodations you will be dealing with, and possibly providing. These are *personal accommodations* and *environmental accommodations*.

Personal accommodations are those you will give to or do specifically with your child, but they will not affect others within the activity. Remember our "screaming at the pool" example from the previous chapter? A dry bathing suit, dry pool shoes, or a piggyback ride to dryer ground would all personally accommodate the child. A set of headphones for loud sounds, a fidget toy, or chewy candy for inappropriate movements or vocalizations are also personal accommodations. Bringing special food to a birthday party, playdate, or picnic would be considered a personal accommodation.

Environmental accommodations affect all of the participants within the activity's environment. Singing the "Happy Birthday" song in whisper voices, or leaving the lights slightly on at the community movie theater during a movie are environmental accommodations. Teaching some simple signs to all of the participants in an activity so that peers can communicate with your child would be an environmental accommodation.

Both personal and environmental accommodations are available to you and your child; you just need to learn to (**A**) accommodate for success, prior to the activity or event.

Accommodating Social Events

Accommodating social events both in and outside of your home will take some preplanning, and possibly a few phone calls. By noting and highlighting the sensory, communicative, skill level, stamina, and food issues your child may face during the activity, you will be able to accommodate your child and fulfill her needs so that she will be more able to self-regulate and interact.

I will give you several examples of how children have been accommodated during recreational activities and family events:

- The coach at a community soccer camp came up with a strategy to help a participant with autism refrain from running rampant on the field—chasing and picking up and taking the ball. He had cones set up on the field in a zigzag pattern, all the way down to the goal. Team members would each stand at a cone and the child with autism was taught to stand at his cone and kick the ball to the "next" cone. They gradually reduced the number of cones, and later had the boy stand at the cone closest to the goal, and when the ball was kicked to him, he would try to kick the ball to the "next" cone—which was the goalie (the cone near the goalie was his visual marker). When this boy kicked a ball past the goalie (which I was told was quite a few times), he was enthusiastically high-fived by the entire soccer team—including the goalie. The boy's parents intend to keep their son in soccer because he seems to really enjoy it, and they are going to request the same coach in the fall.

This boy was accommodated by adding structure and visual markers.

- One family wanted to bring their typical child to Friendly's restaurant for a birthday dinner, but they would have to accommodate their child with autism so that the evening would not be ruined. Usually they would leave their autistic son with a sitter, but his sister insisted he come this time. This child's mother called Friendly's ahead of time, and arranged to have a booth saved in a quieter area—away from the commotion near the front door and the kitchen. During the phone call, the mother also asked that they be warned ahead of time if the waiters or waitresses would be singing "Happy Birthday" to anyone in the restaurant (which involves loud singing and clapping), and asked to have no loud singing or clapping for their daughter—they decided instead to have waiters and waitresses quietly bring over candles and balloons. A backpack of preferred objects and snacks were packed, including a portable DVD player with a favorite video and headphones.

The mother later reported to me that she could not believe how smoothly the dinner went. Their autistic son liked being secluded in the inside corner of the booth, and enjoyed his video while snacking on pretzel sticks. He even attended and seemed intrigued with the balloons and ice cream. (I can't forget to mention that one of the waiters went over to this family and told them he had a brother with autism. This particular waiter offered to do anything or help in any way they needed.)

This autistic child was accommodated with a preferred location and preferred objects and snacks to deflect him from sensory discomforts. The preferred objects and snacks and enclosed seating position helped him to self-regulate through the dinner.

- A community pool made an accommodation for an autistic little girl who refused to get into the water near other children. She would tantrum when brought near the swimming class she was supposed to be a part of. To accommodate her issue, the director at the pool agreed to begin teaching her independently, but *near* the class. Slowly, this little girl calmed and would learn next to the class without issue. Near the end of the session, this girl joined the class with the director standing nearby. If the session had lasted longer, both the director and mother feel, the director could have faded herself out completely.

- One boy with autism was put into an after-school music enrichment class because his parents noticed he had a talent and interest in music. The activity was unsuccessful at first—he would try to bolt and would sometimes yell "No!" over and over. After talking with the mother, the music instructor implemented an immediate snack for all of the kids upon arrival, and she made some music centers and situated them around the room. This boy was given a choice board, made just for him, so he could show his preference of activities. He was also asked to bring in his favorite electronic keyboard from home to show the others—which he did (though he did not want others to touch it).

• One family liked to bring their twins to story hour at their local library, but their autistic twin was extremely distracting, with his vocalizations and constant movement. Other children would move far away from him out of frustration from either being bumped, touched, or kicked. In a conversation with their child's occupational therapist, it was mentioned that their son probably needed some support while sitting—he possibly was not able to sustain an upright position while sitting on the floor. The mother called the library and asked if they would mind if she brought in a special chair. The librarian mentioned they had some bean bag chairs, so they agreed to give one a try. The mother also brought some chewy fruit bites for some "quiet snacking" at the next reading. With the beanbag chair and the chewy bites, this little boy was able to listen to the story, and look around at the other children without inappropriately disturbing them. It was a much more successful experience with just the change in seating and the chewy snack. This boy was accommodated with a physical support and a sensory support (the chewing can be calming for many kids).

Help from the Community

You may be able to provide your child with some personal accommodations on your own, but as you get out more, you will often find yourself in the position of simply not having control over key elements. Before contacting and eliciting the help of others, take a moment and determine what environmental changes you will need to ask for. What environmental elements, when added or subtracted, will help your child?

When you are clear about what to ask for, go ahead and give different venues a call. Most of the time, people will try to make the accommodations you request, so let them know exactly what you need and why it will be helpful. It is harder for staff or hosts to think of and implement accommodations on their own if they do not have prior experience with autistic or special needs kids. The husband of a friend of mine mentioned to me recently that he had no idea he could make these things (accommodations) happen for his son. He said it's really great knowing you can make a big difference for your kid by just asking.

Rest assured, though, that the law is on your side. According to the Americans with Disabilities Act (ADA) PL 101-336, reasonable accommodations must be made by all private, public, and nonprofit agencies that serve the public through recreation, to ensure that those with a disability are not discriminated against. Recreational venues, though, will not be able to accommodate in ways that could put others at risk, for instance, turning off alarms, or refraining from following safety protocols such as blowing whistles at pools and beaches.

It's your child's right to be accommodated. So go for it, and ask for what your child needs.

Action Step for the **A** in I.D.E.**A**.L.: Environmental Addition and Subtraction

I would like you to do an exercise to practice thinking about the types of accommodations your child may need in social activities and outings.

First, choose an upcoming social activity or event (or choose an activity possibility), and check off the issues you expect may come up for your child:

_____ Sensory issues

_____ Communicative issues

_____ Cognitive and comprehension issues

_____ Stamina and fatigue issues

_____ Physical and motor issues

_____ Food allergy and sensitivity issues

Now for each item you have checked off, we are going to do a little *environmental addition* (+) *and subtraction* (−) exercise. Think about the categories you have checked above. For those areas, think about whether you would want to *add* (+) something to the environment (like a preferred object) or *subtract* (−) something from the environment (like bright lighting) to help your child feel at ease. Maybe you would need to do both. Right now, go through the list, and circle the addition signs (+) for those areas you would need to add something or bring something special for your child, and circle the subtraction signs (−) for those areas you would need to eliminate something that causes your child stress.

SENSORY ISSUES

+ _____

− _____

COMMUNICATIVE ISSUES

+ _____

− _____

COGNITIVE AND COMPREHENSION ISSUES

+ _____

− _____

STAMINA AND FATIGUE ISSUES

+ _____

− _____

PHYSICAL AND MOTOR ISSUES

+ _____

− _____

FOOD ALLERGY AND SENSITIVITY ISSUES

+ _____

− _____

Now, for all of the addition (+) and subtraction (−) signs circled, see if you can come up with an accommodation that would help your child self-regulate or participate despite his or her issues. This may take a little time at first, but I promise you, with practice, you will become very quick with this step.

The last step of this exercise is to mark each of your accommodations with either a **P** (for a personal accommodation that you may have access to or bring from home) or an **E** (for an environmental accommodation that you may need to reach out to others for or make phone calls for).

Look at what you have listed. Will these accommodations make the difference for your child? I hope so.

By brainstorming accommodations that can aid in your child's success, you have completed the fourth step in the I.D.E.A.L. process.

CHAPTER 10

■ ■ ■

I.D.E.A.L.

L: List the Activity Components Visually

First we stick on the pictures. You have to make sure they're in
order . . . of what she has to do. See? Look. She can see what she
has to do . . . you could make it so she can see the entire day
before you do any of it.

—*LASHANDA*, age nine,
friend of Crystal, who has Fragile X syndrome

Seeing the components of upcoming activities on visual lists
or charts can help calm and organize children with autism.
Higher-functioning kids may only need to see written words
visually, while others may find words paired with pictures easier
to understand. Other children may need a very realistic pictorial
representation of each task in sequential order to reap the ben-
efits of supplementary visuals.

Most parents find that making some sort of visual schedule

helps their kids immensely in social situations and activities, and many have found ways to incorporate reinforcements directly onto the visual schedules. This helps children to clearly see "where they are" within the planned tasks and activities, as well as when they will receive their reinforcements or rewards (preferred objects or activities). There is a distinct possibility that it will benefit your child if you *visually* represent tasks, and visually represent important rules and safety lessons. The ability to follow rules and directions is very important for later assimilation and independence.

Visual Input and Autism

When I speak about listing activities visually, many often assume that I recommend this because "autistic kids are visual learners." I, personally, do *not* believe that all children with autism are visual learners. I also do not think all children with autism think in pictures. In addition, there is a difference in using visuals as communicative tools for greater understanding, and teaching through visuals. When children are "learning" new skills, they are expected to "remember" the new skills. For instance, some children with autism commit new skills to memory through auditory repetition. Many children with autism have excellent auditory ability and a good memory for sound, patterns, and melodies. Some children learn best with a multisensory approach. But most children with autism have two issues in common: sensory distractibility and language deficits. When autistic children are stressed, language processing, auditory processing, and self-regulation begin to shut down.

The visuals on visual schedules and visual guides are fleeting pieces of knowledge—and may not be "memorized." Children who really are visual learners may be able to commit to memory certain visual guides, but whether the children are visual learners or not, listing components of activities visually, which may, for some children be visual words, helps children by giving them a known pattern of what's to come. It also gives them a focus to help organize themselves, and a tool for understanding when other modes are caving.

Visuals work often, but not always. There is a good chance that they can help support your child's individual issues when among others. It may take a little experimentation to find the right visual schedule presentation for your individual child.

Visual Schedules

Visual schedules are personal tools that use a sequence of pictures or words (or both) to tell a child what will be occurring or what actions need to be taken. Children with autism are often prompted to look at the visual schedules provided for them, but as the use of the tool becomes more automatic, and is understood by the child, many autistic kids begin to use their schedules independently— sometimes with just the prompt to check their schedule.

Visual schedules are used to:

- Calm children, and reduce their anxiety about what's to come.

- Help organize children.

- Help children to independently perform common activities of daily living.

- Show children when breaks and transitions will be occurring.

- Increase comprehension of activities.

- Remind children of behavioral expectations.

- Remind children to interact during certain periods.

- Show changes in plans.

There is no one way to set up a visual schedule, but all visual schedules have an ordered sequence of visual steps.

Since kids with autism are quite different and at different cognitive and communicative levels, there are many different ways to level visual schedules so that they can have one that is just right for them. Some children may have great difficulty attending to any concrete matter, and may need to begin with a sequence of objects, called an *object schedule*. An object schedule is a "pre–visual schedule" that uses objects that the child can touch and hold (to gain his attention). Each object represents the activity to go to. If parents begin to implement an object schedule with their children, they should begin to use the starter words for sequencing, which are "first . . . " and "then . . . " As children become more familiar with the meaning of being handed an object, and the vocabulary of sequencing, parents can begin to use visuals of the exact objects used in the object schedule to make a child's first visual schedule.

Visual schedules may be made up of sequences of photos, online pictures, PECS pictures, line drawings, words, or sentences. It is important that the schedule be a sequence of pictures, words, or sentences your child recognizes.

When entering into social activities and events with your child, you can make a visual schedule directly from your activity task analysis. You already know how to list in sequential order the steps of an activity or task. Making this list visual will not be a difficult task for you. It is worth the little bit of time and trouble locating pictures or writing out words. Participating without a visual schedule, and without knowing or remembering what is to come, may be a difficult task for your child.

Visual schedules may be arranged from left to right, or they may be arranged from top to bottom. Whichever you choose, try to make sure that the sequence you use is visually clear and not cluttered. Some children can only tolerate looking at one to three pictures on a board or paper. Children can be easily distracted when there is too much in their visual field. It may take a little experimentation to find a visual schedule that works well for your child, but once you find something that works, it can help open up many doors to independence, since it can be used in so many ways.

Visual schedules can be made using clipboards, write-on wipe-off boards, laminated pieces of cardboard or construction paper, or small pieces of poster board. Velcro is often used in squares or strips to hold the sequences of pictures or words. Little "libraries" of pictures and words are often attached and carried with the visual schedule. Parents usually keep the extra words and pictures in pencil cases, zip-top sandwich bags, or envelopes. Some like to stick the extra pictures and words to Velcro on the backside of the visual schedule.

Incorporating Reinforcements and Rewards Visually

Your child will need positive reinforcements for doing the right thing, and for making efforts that you want to encourage. The visual schedule can help keep your child in tune with how she is doing, as you stick on or draw visual checks, stars, smiley faces, or tokens. It is helpful to have a picture depicting the preferred object or activity your child is "working for" or earning right on the visual schedule. Some like to put a check or star next to each task as it is completed. Others like to put a line of Velcro next to the picture of the reward so that the child can earn a certain number of tokens according to her own individual schedules of reinforcement.

Using Visuals for Activities and Events

Within social activities and events, it is natural not to want to be constantly on your child's heels pointing to visual schedules, or pulling out new task lists with every showing of an interest or intent. And your child should not be stifled from the freedom to initiate an interaction or show an interest when it is not on "the schedule." As you begin to use these tools, however, the "how much" and the "ebb and flow" of when to intervene (and when to not intervene) reveal themselves and come into better focus. Depending on the individual children, some may need a visual schedule simply for a basic knowledge of what is to come. Other kids really *do* need tasks broken down and visually "explained." The children who require higher amounts of interventions and the children who have greater needs will slowly gain independence and need lesser amounts of steps, prompts, and guidance in the future.

Using Visuals for Rules and Safety

The codes of conduct, and varying expectations in the many different social venues and situations we find ourselves in, can be very confusing for children with autism. The rules (and freedom) of movement, behavior, and volume are very different on the playground, at Grandma's, and at the local church.

One fun way to help prime children and prepare them for these typically unspoken rules of behavior is to visually use preferred objects and characters on rule lists. Another option (for our auditory learners) is to speak like a preferred character (if you have the talent) and recite the rule list (and then check for understanding).

I like to print out a preferred character picture from an online site (one student of mine becomes *very* attentive when he sees "Dark Batman") and paste it to the top of a list of simple concrete rules. It is amazing to see the heightened level of attending when a favorite character is somehow involved.

A Note About Visual Schedules

The visual schedule is the tool your child will use when he or she is at the actual activity or event. It is all right to show your child the visual schedule as you "introduce" the activity using "social stories," picture walks, et cetera, but please do not leave the visual schedule out to be played with. You can bring it out again and again if your child needs another look, but be relatively brief and matter-of-fact with your reviewing of the tasks. Previewing and priming your child can last one day, or two weeks. You will have to find what works best for your child's personality. Some children feel a lot of anxiety, even when it is positive excitement, and find it hard to sleep—which, as you can imagine, can become an issue over several days. Through trial and error, or through your gut feeling, you will find what works best for your child.

Action Step for the **L** in I.D.E.A.**L**.

I would like you to choose an activity or task (you may do this in your home), and create a visual schedule for your child. Include three to five sequential steps, and depending on your child's level and abilities, choose to use pictures, words, or both. Make your visual schedule using paper or cardboard—whatever you are comfortable with. You may use a previously written task analysis, if you wish.

Before using the visual schedule with your child, look at it carefully. Would your child attend to the way it looks? Look at the background (color, et cetera) and the foreground (how noticeable the pictures and words are, how they look against the background, et cetera) and take note of any adjustments you think of that would help your child to attend to the tasks.

Next, show the visual schedule to your child, and let your child make a (verbal, gestural, or visual) choice of a reward to work for. Prompt him or her to begin using the visual schedule, and reprompt your child with each step, if needed. Was your child able to understand that he or she would be rewarded after completing the series of tasks? What changes would you make to your original first schedule?

By listing the activity tasks visually for your child, you have completed the fifth step in the I.D.E.A.L. process.

The following is an I.D.E.A.L. template and planning sheet that you can use repeatedly when planning for and preparing your child for playdates, outings, and events.

I.D.E.A.L.

I: Introduce the Activity

MODE OF INTRODUCTION (CHECK AT LEAST ONE):

_____ Previsit to environment
_____ Photographic walk

_____ "Social story"
_____ Bubble book or comic strip
_____ Role playing
_____ Video modeling

D: Determine the Tasks Involved

Task: _____

Mark each task step with an **I**—meaning your child can do the step independently, or with a **P**—meaning your child will need to be prompted.

1.

2.

3.

4.

5.

6.

7.

8.

9.

10.

E: Evaluate Your Expectations

Duration: My child will attend from _____a.m./p.m. to _____a.m./p.m.

My child will need _____ (#) breaks.

Personal goals and expectations: _____

_____

_____

A: Accommodate for Success

Do some environmental addition and subtraction. Then mark whether each accommodation is personal or environmental by circling either the **P** or **E**.

SENSORY ISSUES

+ _____ P   E

− _____ P   E

COMMUNICATIVE ISSUES

+ _____ P   E

− _____ P   E

COGNITIVE AND COMPREHENSION ISSUES

+ _____ P   E

− _____ P   E

STAMINA AND FATIGUE ISSUES

+ _____ P   E

− _____ P   E

PHYSICAL AND MOTOR ISSUES

+ _____ P   E

− _____ P   E

FOOD ALLERGY AND SENSITIVITY ISSUES

+ _____ P   E

− _____ P   E

L: List the Activity Components Visually

The visual schedule will list tasks with (check at least one):

_____ Objects (object schedule)

_____ Pictures

_____ Words

_____ Sentences

A schedule of reinforcement will be visually presented: yes_____ no_____

If yes, fill in below:

MY CHILD WILL BE WORKING FOR (LIST SOME PREFERRED OBJECTS AND ACTIVITIES):

_____

_____

_____

Facilitating Social

Opportunities Using

I.D.E.A.L.

CHAPTER 11

■   ■   ■

Playdates

I went to her house. I think it's nice for her to have me as her best friend. She always smiles at me and that makes me . . . want to make her smile again.

—*CAITLIN*, *age seven*,
friend of Morgan, who has autism and epilepsy

The last part of this book is about taking action. We will begin to put all of the tools and information you have gathered thus far to use, as we start to preview and plan social activities and outings for your child using the I.D.E.A.L. system. And we will start with what is the staple of socialization for young children—the playdate.

As we begin to plan playdates for our kids with autism, we will need to think of playdates as we never have before. To help ourselves be better able to prepare our children with autism, we will need to take a *literal* and comprehensive look at the sequence of events that make up a playdate. This means you will be introducing "what a playdate is and looks like" to your child, analyzing the steps involved, setting expectations, accommodating, and visually representing the sequence, so your child will know how to proceed. As you approach parents of potential "friends," you will feel confident knowing you have prepared well. So let's get started.

The Sequential Steps of a Playdate

So, what exactly is a playdate? Usually one child is dropped off at your house, or your child is dropped off at another child's house . . . and the kids play. Right? What would your child do if a friend were "dropped off" to play for two hours? Would you feel comfortable dropping your child off at a friend's house and leaving for a span of time?

We need to think of playdates a little differently for children with autism, and approach each playdate as an opportunity for socialization and fun using a structured (but flexible) plan of sequential events.

If we think of what a playdate may entail sequentially from beginning to end, we can begin to brainstorm activities, locations, durations (amounts of time), breaks needed, and the times of day to have a playdate. Here are three examples of different playdate formats:

FORMAT A

Greeting
Activity
Snack
Good-bye

FORMAT B

Greeting
Activity 1
Activity 2
Snack
Good-bye

FORMAT C

Greeting
Activity 1
Activity 2
Snack
Activity 3
Good-bye

As you look at a format that may work for your child, you can begin to think about durations. How long of an activity would your child tolerate with another? This varies greatly among the kids, and the playmate is also a factor. Some children enjoy or tolerate interactions with certain play friends longer than other play friends, so each playdate will need to be individually planned for.

You may need to guide and prompt each step of the playdate until your child gets the hang of the "scheme," but it is well worth it. Thinking in terms of a playdate format can make it easy for you to plan each sequential step.

The greeting you would like your child to perform, as well as all the activities you plan to do during the playdate, can be primed beforehand, and introduced to your child using one of the introduction techniques beforehand. Maybe after considering your child's unique skills and tolerance levels, the general format for the playdate would look something like this:

Greeting—using partial verbal prompts
Activity 1—shaving cream finger painting at the
      kitchen table
Activity 2—trampoline in the backyard
Snack—cheese crackers and juice
Good-bye—using partial verbal prompts

If your child can tolerate and do a pretty good job of handling these activities, this would be a great playdate to start with. Let's now jump into the I.D.E.A.L. process and prepare for the playdate using this example.

Previewing and Planning a Playdate Using I.D.E.A.L.

- **I**ntroduce the Activity.

- **D**etermine the Tasks Involved.

- **E**valuate Your Expectations.

- **A**ccommodate for Success.

- **L**ist the Activity Components Visually.

First we would want to introduce the activity to your child. Maybe we could write a "social story" about the upcoming playdate, or possibly your child would understand a photographic walk better, where he could see pictures of himself playing with shaving cream, jumping on the trampoline, and eating the preferred snack. Now, even though we may have a playdate format with activities in mind, we still need to determine the tasks involved. This would be a list of tasks that *your child* would have to perform sequentially to be successful. Let's list them here:

PLAYDATE

Say hi to Sam.
Say hi to Sam's mom.
Go sit down at kitchen table.
Pull up sleeves.
Play with shaving cream!
Wash hands in bathroom.
Go outside and jump on trampoline.
Take turns with Sam.
Wash hands in bathroom.
Go sit at kitchen table.
Wait.
Eat snack.
Throw away napkin.
Say good-bye to Sam.
Say good-bye to Sam's mom.

Depending on your own child's level, your task list may be brief or very involved. Just make your best guess as to how involved—you will see from even one use of a task list in an actual social setting whether your child would benefit from a more detailed task list, or a more simplified one.

To evaluate your expectations, look at each step of the task list and determine which of the steps your child can do independently and which will need to be prompted. Then determine the time durations you think each piece of the playdate format will take. You can use the format *or* the task list to determine durations.

In this particular example, I believe the greeting would only be about a minute; the shaving cream activity would probably be about 15 minutes; the trampoline fun would probably be 25 minutes; and the snack would be about 15 minutes. Seeing this, I would call the parent and invite the child (playdate friend) over for 1 hour.

After you have established the parameters of the playdate, you should begin to look at the accommodations your child may need to help maintain his self-regulation. In this particular example, the actual choices of activities may in and of themselves be accommodating—since they are sensory-motor activities. Possibly the activities will help reduce self-stimming behaviors. Maybe you know that your child will need some prompting for turn taking, so you decide to use a timer as an accommodation that you will set for two-minute turns.

Lastly, to prepare for the playdate, list the components visually for your child, using pictures, words, or both. This will help your child to see and understand what will be happening at the beginning, middle, and end of the playdate. It is helpful to use your introduction method for several days to a week before the actual playdate. Your list of components (task list) can be introduced along with the introduction method, or if you do not have it prepared in time, showing it the night before, and the morning of the playdate will be helpful so that there will be some familiarity. If your child shows great interest in the task list, let him look at it for a little while, but then put the list away until the next showing or until the actual playdate. Do not let your child carry the task list around for an extended period of time or begin to play with it.

Pre-Playdate Considerations

Before your child's playdate takes place, there are some "pre-playdate considerations" to reflect on. These would include whom to invite, and whether the playdates' parents will be receptive to and understand your needs for preplanning. (Have you ever felt like you look "neurotic"?) Sometimes it is helpful to review in your mind or on paper what you will say on the telephone or in person as you discuss some of the playdate issues and activities with other parents.

Here is an example of a phone script to use when inviting a playdate (if your child is unable to do this independently) over to your house:

> Hi—this is [*first and last name*]. My child knows your [*son/ daughter*] from [*location*]. My [*son/daughter (name)*] really enjoys playing with your [*son/daughter (name)*], and I was wondering if you and [*possible playdate's name*] would be interested in coming over, just for an hour [*or other time amount*], for a play-date. You are welcome to come and stay. We can have coffee and talk while the kids play.

Often, you will find (and this can be a little disconcerting at times) that parents of children you want to invite already know who your child is, and who you are. This is usually because typical children often have questions that they bring to their parents about children with special needs. Being "known" in your community can be helpful in a way, though too, because you do not have to introduce and educate the other parent about your child's autism during that initial phone call. It is important, though, that if you feel the parent you are calling has not had exposure to your child, and may not know your child has autism, you add to the phone script something like:

> [*Son/daughter's name*] has autism, and I can't tell you how much it means to [*son/daughter's name*] to have [*possible playdate's name*] show [*him/her*] friendship. You have a wonderful [*son/daughter*].

Even if you will be prompting your child, you do not have to establish on the phone or (during the playdate) in person that you will be assisting during Steps 6 and 9. During the playdate, just get up and do the prompting you need to do as it comes.

Another consideration is that you may not be able to control what the playdate does or says—so there will be some unknowns no matter how well you have planned. Typical kids range in intellect levels and behavior, so remember (and accept the challenge) that you will be dealing with *two* kids during the playdate.

Post-Playdate Debriefings

After each playdate your child "hosts" or attends, take a moment to debrief while looking at or thinking about your original I.D.E.A.L. plan. Ask yourself the following questions:

1. What successes did my child experience at the playdate?

2. Was the playdate a good match for my child's abilities?

3. Did my child interact with the playdate friend? (When?)

4. Was the playdate friend someone I would want to pursue for friendship for my child?

5. Am I happy with my choice of introduction to the activity?

6. Was I able to accurately determine the tasks involved?

7. Were my expectations appropriate?

8. Do I want to make note of areas to accommodate better next time?

9. Did my child attend to the visuals I supplied?

Your child's socialization experiences with playdates will not only be learning experiences for your child, but for you, too.

Take a look at some of the experiences other moms have had setting up playdates with I.D.E.A.L. for their children with autism.

Examples of Playdates and the Value of I.D.E.A.L.

I invited a classmate of my son's over. His teacher recommended a child named David, and he really was a sweetheart. I had planned a two-hour playdate because one hour just felt too short to me, and I lived to regret it. I also think initially I overestimated what my son would do independently with this boy. I ended up constantly needing to prompt my son, and had definitely not broken down the activities into clear enough steps. My son's frustration with me trying to get him to keep up with David caused him to run away up to his room around the time David had to leave. During the playdate I was upset with myself briefly for maybe not planning as well as I should have, but I remembered [Laurie LeComer] saying that we learn a lot from that first time.

I use I.D.E.A.L. religiously now and much more carefully, and playdates have been smoother. Though at first I thought "social stories" would work best for my son, I found that the photographic walk helped him much more. So we use that now to introduce what he'll be doing. I keep playdates down to an hour, and sometimes have mini–playdates with neighborhood kids for a half hour at a time. So I definitely have him socializing 1000% more than before I knew of a good way to do it.

I learned my expectations were a little off, but I am better with that now, and can better anticipate what he'll be able to take on when a friend is over, and I feel no guilt now about accommodating if I have to. I've told kids to speak quietly around my son, and to not rush around, yell, or scream, and I've put headphones on my son's ears when it's been his turn on the computer, and a friend or neighbor is squealing out loud around him.

I always now list the parts of the playdate visually. I just use pictures, and I check them off or have my son check them off as we go. I feel very good about this step of now having playdates. I see his comfort growing—it's just one of the things he does now. It's almost expected now.

I thought I.D.E.A.L made sense when I saw the different steps, and I liked going through the preparation steps. I felt like we had a pretty good handle on preparing our son for seeing friends and having friends over. We had been using "social stories" for some time, and would bring things with us, but that was pretty much the extent of our preparation before I.D.E.A.L.

I think I.D.E.A.L. has helped us in a couple ways—probably different from most of the others trying I.D.E.A.L. for the first time. When I did a playdate task analysis, I realized that my son really could do a lot of tasks independently—especially when they are broken down into little steps. There were places I would need to give reminders, but it dawned on me that I had been taking over so-to-speak and not waiting for or allowing him to do what he really could do. Another "moment" I had while using I.D.E.A.L. was after the fact in the debriefing questions part—I realized that my friend's son who I used often as a play partner was probably not the best match, and probably not even a good role model for a friend for my son. He would tease some, and was not well behaved. I think I used him as a play partner because his mom is a friend of mine, so it was easy for me to arrange. After realizing this, I did contact my son's special education teacher and speech therapist for friend recommendations, and I have three possibilities to call.

For me, now that I have used I.D.E.A.L., the order is so easy to remember, you find yourself just naturally going through the steps in your head, and I find that I am probably more prepared even for little comings and goings than before.

I'm embarrassed to say that using I.D.E.A.L. was probably the first time I preplanned and really thought through my child's social encounters with other kids. In Sarah's school she uses a visual activity chart, but I never used one in our house until recently—after seeing how interested she was in everything visual I showed her. Sarah can read a little, so I put pictures and words on the activity schedule. She spent so much time looking at it and became so obsessed with it that she wanted to stick to the exact playdate schedule—to the "T." For a time there, I just stood and watched her go. Her friend even got a kick out of it because she was usually not forward with anyone at school. She knew what came first, and next, and dragged her friend—in a good way—with her from one activity to the next. She seemed almost inspired by the activity list. At previous playdates, it was common for Sarah to become frustrated and lie down on the floor, but this didn't happen with the preplanning. I had her favorite soda ready and waiting in the fridge for her and her friend to share if I saw any signs of needing a break. I liked what the preplanning did for Sarah, and from looking at the I.D.E.A.L. steps, I can see how it may help others.

My son has moderate to severe autism, so socializing is very difficult for him, and he really needs support from an adult no matter where he is. Using I.D.E.A.L. showed me that it is okay to begin with just a half hour for a playdate, or maybe even a twenty-minute playdate. I like that no matter the difficulties your child faces, you can really look at them and make decisions that won't hurt your child, and will really in the end benefit your child. My son loves to eat, so I made small playdates of making cookies. He understands that when we mix batter and add ingredients, cookies will be coming! My son will literally watch them bake through the window of the oven—but a friend keeps him company while he watches. I see him look at his friends sometimes—he knows he is with and involved with another during the baking. He loves the cookies, and his friends always do, too. It is motivating to him and the boys that come over—because the results are so yummy! Bravo to using I.D.E.A.L.!

CHAPTER 12

■   ■   ■

Birthday Parties

I think if I invite him to my birthday party, he might see it's fun,
and then he could be able to have his own birthday parties.

—*DREW, age five,*
friend of Daniel, who has autism

The excitement of birthday parties can cause even the most typical of kids to feel overwhelmed, but for kids with autism, the elevated sensory experience may cause them to completely lose their composure. The noise level and abundant visual stimulation may cause kids to shut down or act out with aggression. Once a child is overstimulated, it is often hard to calm him down until he is removed from the environment. By using the I.D.E.A.L. system, you will be able to take preventative action and make party experiences thought-out learning opportunities, tailor-made for your child's unique characteristics and ability level.

Just like with playdates, you will analyze what makes up a

birthday party and will introduce the activity to your child beforehand in a mode that works best for him. Again, the tasks involved will be broken down, including the length of each task, so that you can have realistic expectations about your child's participation, and know what your child will be able to do independently and what he will need assistance with. When prepping for birthday parties, you may be able to set up accommodations by yourself, or you may need to enlist other parents to help you. Birthday party tasks can be listed visually for your child on his visual schedule, or you can put visuals on a portable notebook or an easy-to-carry note card.

Your child should have some comforting tools throughout every birthday event. So, let's get started and look more closely at the steps involved in attending or having a birthday party.

The Sequential Steps of a Birthday Party

Birthday parties can be a little more difficult to navigate than playdates, since the autistic chld must cope with increased sensory input owing to the larger numbers of kids and people. There is also usually a palpable heightened anxiety of those who are either attending or running the party.

I recommend that your child have a point person, no matter whether it is a party outside of the house, or within your own house, who will model "calm" and be available to your child at all times. Maybe this will be you when attending a party outside your home, but if you are hosting a birthday party in your own home, for either your child, a sibling, or a family member, and are in charge of most of the activities, your child with autism will need a specific person available to her—to help her when needed, or to guide her. That someone should be able to observe your child for signs of the need for interference or a break. This could be a spouse, a sibling, a grandparent, or a babysitter. It is important to establish who this person will be beforehand, so you can let your child know when you introduce the activity in "social stories," or photographic walks, whom to go to and whom to take direction from. For best results, this person should be someone your child already knows well.

Birthday parties may take place at friends' houses, but they are increasingly out in the community, at malls, parks, and recreational venues. It is always helpful to visit these special party venues so that you can better prepare your child using I.D.E.A.L. And with invitations to birthday parties sometimes being few and far between, when one does arrive, it is important to really take a moment and think about ways your child can be prepared and primed to attend—at least for a portion.

Upon entering any birthday party, there is such an immediate rush of sensory stimuli that getting over that initial hurdle of entering with one's self-regulation and composure intact can be considered a success.

Let's look at some examples of birthday party formats. I am going to use the term "birthday table" to represent the step when the partygoers gather at a table, light candles, sing, and have cake.

FORMAT A

Initial entering experience
Greeting
Activity
Birthday table
Opening of presents
Good-bye

FORMAT B

Initial entering experience
Greeting
Activity 1
Food table
Activity 2
Birthday table
Opening of presents
Good-bye

FORMAT C

Initial entering experience
Activity 1
Activity 2
Birthday table
Activity 3
Opening of presents
Good-bye

Some children do not open presents at their parties, and some have lunches or dinners included with their parties, so there is a lot of variation. These formats are visually depicted to give you a linear and literal way of looking at the process and movement of typical birthday parties. It is important to look at a birthday party in this way because the initial entering and then the movement usually directed to an activity may not be a motivating sequence of events for children with autism. This is why when you look at these formats, and think about your own child, look at what may occur in what order. Would your child have a greater chance of success with the peers at the party if he or she entered at a time when the party was moving directly to food or the birthday table? Would your child do better coming for an ending activity and watching the presents being opened long after the hoopla of the birthday table? There is no one right way, and you should not feel pressured to make your child try to deal with an extended time span among such intense stimuli if he or she is simply not ready to handle it. Possibly your child could handle an accommodated chunk. By going through the steps of I.D.E.A.L., you will have a good idea of where to start.

Previewing and Planning a Birthday Party Using I.D.E.A.L.

- **I**ntroduce the Activity.

- **D**etermine the Tasks Involved.

- **E**valuate Your Expectations.

- **A**ccommodate for Success.

- **L**ist the Activity Components Visually.

As with the playdate, you will need to introduce the upcoming birthday party to your child in a mode your child will understand. Have you found a mode that works best for your child as you've set up playdates? Of the families I work with, the photographic walks and the "social stories" are the most popular options, but remember, all of the kids are very individual from one another, so use what works best for your child.

Determining the tasks involved can be a little tricky, especially if the birthday party is not one that you are hosting. Thank goodness for those RSVP phone numbers at the bottom of those birthday invitations! When you pick up the phone and RSVP, let the parents know how helpful it would be to you and your child to know the plan of events beforehand. Be open about your child needing to see the different steps to successfully attend, or come forth with your anticipation of only being able to attend for a chunk of time. If your child was invited, they want him to come. Period. Your extra preparation will make the party a more enjoyable experience for all.

Let's say your child was invited to a birthday party at a bowling alley. Though you may know the format of the party, you should determine the tasks involved—from your child's eyes and standpoint. A task list may look something like this:

BOWLING PARTY

Get in car.
Listen to music CD.
Get out of car.
Walk with Mom into bowling alley.
Hold present.
Walk to Jason.
Say, "Happy Birthday, Jason!"
Give Jason present.
Walk to seat.
Watch bowling.
On my turn—pick up bowling ball.
Roll ball down floor to pins.
Sit down.
(A sequence of steps may repeat as child has several
turns.)
Walk to birthday table.
Sit down.

(Put on my headphones and listen to CD.)

Eat snack (brought from home if can't eat cake).

Give headphones to Mom.

Walk to seat.

Watch bowling.

On my turn—pick up bowling ball.

Roll ball down floor to pins.

Sit down.

Go to presents table.

Sit down.

Look at Jason open presents.

Go to Jason.

Say, "Bye. See you at school!"

Walk with Mom to car.

Get in car.

Listen to music CD.

Get out of car.

Go to bathroom at home.

If your child understands his visual task list, there is a good chance he will be able to successfully navigate the party, and these steps in sequential order. Some of these steps your child may be able to perform independently, and some of them may need to be assisted, so you should go through each task and mark whether, **I**—your child can do the step independently, or **P**—your child will need prompts.

Next, you need to evaluate your expectations. Seeing what your child can and can't do independently is helpful, but you need to make a good decision about the duration your child can successfully handle. Perhaps after some careful consideration, you decide your child will only be able to handle a chunk of the party so you decide to skip the later part. Your child's task list for the party may now be a more manageable and realistic series of tasks that look like this:

BOWLING PARTY

Walk to Jason.
Say, "Happy Birthday, Jason!"
Give Jason present.
Walk to seat.
Watch bowling.
On my turn—pick up bowling ball.
Roll ball down floor to pins.
Sit down.
(A sequence of steps may repeat as child has several
        turns.)
Walk to birthday table.
Sit down.
(Put on my headphones and listen to CD.)
Snack (brought from home if can't eat cake).
Give headphones to Mom.
Go to Jason.
Say, "Bye. See you at school!"
Walk with Mom to car.
Get in car.
Listen to music CD.
Get out of car.
Go to bathroom at home.

You have probably noticed a few accommodations, such as the headphones, listed within the task list. You will find that you will begin to include accommodations you know are needed, naturally—even before you reach the step where a careful focus is taken on accommodating. To accommodate for success, you shortened the party to ensure greater (even if brief) participation Listening to a CD in the car and listening to a CD with head-phones at the party are accommodations to help with sensory needs. The snack brought from home is an accommodation—your child may be on a special diet and not be able to eat typical "birthday food." All these accommodations are personal accom-modations and do not affect the experience of the other attend-ees at the party. They are also easy to bring, do, and are perfect small allowances to help your child self-regulate and remain rea-sonably comfortable.

Lastly, in preparation for the birthday party, you will need to list the activity components visually for your child. Use what you have found works best—just words, or pictures, or a combina-tion of both—these visuals are solely to help your child navigate the birthday party and enjoy the experience.

Pre–Birthday Party Considerations

When preparing your child to attend a birthday party or for a birthday party in your home, the ambience of the environment will need to be carefully considered. As the number of attendees grows, a feeling of commotion may also grow, so you need to know a little bit about the numbers, and the environmental stimuli—because it will all come crashing down on your child's senses. If you are in control, and having the party, you can keep the numbers down, and possibly keep certain personalities in check by either hiring extra help, or asking other family members to be watchful and to help when necessary. You can also let other children know what your expectations are for them in your environment. Keep the time allotted down to an amount that is doable for your child. Though your child's birthday party may seem a little shorter than usual to others, it may seem like the most successful party yet to your child.

Post–Birthday Party Debriefings

After each birthday party your child has or attends, take a minute and ask yourself the following questions:

1. What successes did my child experience at the birthday party?

2. Were the party activities enjoyed by my child?

3. Which activities at the party were my child's "preferred activities"?

4. Could the birthday boy or girl be a potential friend for my child (if it's a peer's birthday)?

5. Am I happy with my choice of introduction for the birthday party?

6. Was I able to accurately determine the tasks involved?

7. Were my expectations appropriate?

8. Do I want to make note of areas to accommodate better next time?

9. Did my child attend to the visuals I supplied?

With each party you have or with each party your child attends, you will keep learning more about the little duration changes and accommodations that will make big, positive differences for your child.

Let's take a look at some birthday party experiences other moms have had with their children with autism.

Examples of Birthday Parties and the Value of I.D.E.A.L.

I went through the steps of I.D.E.A.L. to give my son a birthday party in our house. It was an interesting adventure for me because it was the first time we—my husband and I—gave Daniel a party where friends from school were invited. We always just had a family party with his favorite foods, presents, and cake. So I found that the "social story" seemed to work really well. He wanted me to read it to him several times a day, so I think he was excited about the whole thing. Because the party was at our house, I basically decorated the backyard, and chose a two-activity party format in which the first activity would be playing in the backyard, and the second activity would be putting Daniel's favorite cartoon movie onto the big-screen TV. I decided to have pizza and then cake in between the two activities.

Well, things were going well, but what I didn't plan for was my husband being held up when he went out to pick up the pizza. So what I decided to do was have the cake. I thought we could just dig into the pizza when my husband arrived with it. Well, I shouldn't have done this—because Daniel had a meltdown because he knew that the pizza was supposed to come first according to the order we had planned.

I felt really bad because everything was going so well, and he was with the other kids, and I hadn't even realized how important that visual chart was to him. He really knew and had absorbed what we would be doing and when.

In the corner of my mind, I remembered that section about what to do if there was a sudden change in plans, and I sat on the floor with Daniel and quickly wrote a new "social story" for him, and it worked! We calmly changed the picture order on the visual schedule. My husband walked in a few minutes later and Daniel went right up to him, letting him know of the changes and showing him the "revised" visual chart.

It really just touched my heart how communicative he was and how he took charge in a way when he felt it was important for us and for the party. I.D.E.A.L. guided me, and continues to guide me—it is especially wonderful at those times I am frazzled and too tired to think of everything that needs to be thought of.

I planned a birthday party for our son at our YMCA pool and did a lot of preplanning using I.D.E.A.L., where in the process, I came up with the idea of hiring Jamey's swim instructor for an hour to help me out so that I could do the welcoming and set up the cake and favors in the party room. I had to call beforehand and do a lot of talking to get what I needed, but I knew what I needed—it was really clear after doing the task analysis and the environmental addition and subtraction exercise.

Jamey does not transition well and has a difficult time with people he doesn't know, so one day when I was talking with his instructor, we came up with the accommodation where when it would be time for cake, Jamey would remain with her (his instructor) in the pool while all of the other kids would get out of the pool, go to the locker room, where my husband and I would be—and then go sit down at the party table. The swim instructor would get Jamey out as they do at his lesson, and she would dry him and bring him to the room after everyone was seated and not running around. Well this, coupled with the Pokemon plates, which Jamey noticed right away—my own accommodation to make him happy—worked great! I am thrilled, and I thank you.

I decided to accept an invitation for a birthday party where I would be bringing my son to a miniature golf pizza party. I probably would not have gone but needed a good excuse to try out I.D.E.A.L. We have not been big on attending active places. I did not bring him for the entire party, but I was definitely pleased with how the hour we were there went. We arrived with our activity chart in hand during the pizza-eating time. My son does not like cake, but he did eat several pieces of pizza. I found myself pleasantly surprised by the kids at the party. During the pizza, several kids tried to engage with my son, and were very nice with him. After the pizza, I showed where we were on the activity chart, and we planned to watch the golf. One of the other boys helped him try to putt.

Things were going well, and I wanted to exit while things were going well—so yes, it got us out, and we had a nice hour out. I'm feeling good about "the hour," too. Right now, it seems like it would be a good idea to do weekly hour mini-get-togethers with others. That one experience had an impact on me. I did not expect him to do as well as he did.

CHAPTER 13

■ ■ ■

Family Holiday Gatherings

I wish my family could stay together at Christmas and Thanksgiving and other times. My mom always has to stay home or leave with my brother. So it's always just me and my dad at my grandmother's or something.

—NATALIE, age nine,

little sister to Trevor, who has Angelman syndrome with autism

---

Family holiday gatherings hold many challenges for kids with autism, but they also offer many opportunities for true engagement and relating to others. Many parents that I work with tell me how difficult it is to stay connected to their relatives, friends, and religious traditions. Oftentimes, any excitement or changes in routine are avoided to keep from escalating undesirable behaviors in their children.

As with playdates and birthday parties, previewing and planning with I.D.E.A.L. can enable you to continue sharing your traditions and celebrations. Little will be left to the imagination as you go through the five steps and plan exactly how your child will be included and involved. As with other events, you will discern where your child can act independently, and where he will need assistance. By drawing from the numerous sensory and behavioral strategies in this book, you will also be able to accommodate in ways that will make the experience more comfortable for your child. You may find that visual schedules help your child to enter and tolerate family celebrations better, and you may be surprised by unexpected successes, such as seeing your child show interest in others, or seeing your child try new games or foods. In order to understand further how to fit the pieces of a plan together for a successful holiday experience, we need to look at family holiday gatherings in a concrete and literal way. I hope, as you read this chapter, that you will feel confident and excited about your future family celebrations. And with practice, your child, too, can learn to look forward to certain holiday traditions with wonder and excitement.

The Sequential Steps of a Family Holiday Gathering

Many of our holidays are a feast for the senses, but for children with autism, finding the joy when there are overwhelming sensory stimuli around every corner can be challenging. Children with autism often like to "know" their territories, and "know" their daily routines, but at holiday gatherings and even at holiday times, even little things like decorations can throw them off. Seeing objects placed where they usually are not and having to wear clothing that is new or not of the "everyday feel" can be unsettling and disturbing to sensitive kids. Holiday gatherings usually involve an even higher level of interacting than birthday parties, and autistic kids may find themselves being prodded and prompted to look more, say more, and possibly give more than they really can when under stress. Kissing, hugging, and touching, which all regularly occur at family holiday gatherings, can be especially uncomfortable for children with autism, and many parents have told stories of their kids losing control upon just entering holiday events—because of the kissing and hugging. If your child would do better avoiding this step, you should note it as you go through the steps of I.D.E.A.L.

Other parents have mentioned how hard it can be to keep their kids' hands out of the food that is put out for guests, or they have told stories of their kids taking and eating so much that they end up vomiting. This issue could be noted and accommodated as you prepare with I.D.E.A.L. If you let the host or hostess know of this possibility beforehand, they could plan for an alternative method of serving food to guests. This would be an environmental accommodation because it would affect all of those attending the function, but no one except the host or hostess would even know there had been a change.

Let's now look at some examples of holiday gathering formats.

FORMAT A

Initial entering experience
Greetings
Meal
Unstructured interacting
Good-byes

FORMAT B

Initial entering experience
Greetings
Unstructured interacting
Meal
Unstructured interacting
Good-byes

FORMAT C

Initial entering experience
Greetings
Activity
Meal
Unstructured interacting
Good-byes

You may have noticed that the sample formats of family holiday gatherings rely heavily on unstructured interacting—even when the host and hostess have decorated, are making the rounds, and have cooked up a lovely gourmet meal. This makes holiday gatherings a hotbed for inappropriate behaviors, because children with autism are not usually at their best during unstructured time periods. Does this mean you should not bring your child to family holiday gatherings? Absolutely not! This means you will give those unstructured periods of time a structure. By planning with I.D.E.A.L., you will plan and bring whatever it is your child needs to feel happily busy and content during those periods. You may need some accommodations, and you may need to designate a quiet room your child can go to—even if it is just for a chunk in the beginning. It is important to maintain your family connections, and to celebrate your traditions and holidays.

Previewing and Planning a Family Holiday Gathering Using I.D.E.A.L.

- **I**ntroduce the Activity.

- **D**etermine the Tasks Involved.

- **E**valuate Your Expectations.

- **A**ccommodate for Success.

- **L**ist the Activity Components Visually.

You will begin to get ready for your holiday gathering by choosing a way to introduce the activity or event to your child. Sometimes it's fun to have the host or hostess e-mail you pictures of their house and some special decorations they have out. Your child may enjoy previewing the decorations, and then pointing them out to you at the actual event. Again, visiting beforehand, taking a photographic walk, or reviewing a "social story" can help your child prepare. If the holiday party will be in your own home, and you are worried about your child's reaction to the change in familiar scenery, you can show your child some magazine pictures of decorated living rooms and stairwells, and leave some decorations out for a couple days—just lying around. See if your child tries to imitate the magazine picture on his or her own, or encourage your child to help you make a room look like the magazine picture.

Another introductory activity you may want to consider for family holiday gatherings is to preview the faces and names of the people your child will see at the event. This will take pre-planning, because you will need recent pictures of family and friends to review with your child. Again, this is just a step in the I.D.E.A.L. process.

Once the activity is introduced to your child, you will need to determine the tasks involved, and if you are attending a holiday gathering elsewhere, a phone call may be needed to find out the plan of events, so that you can be accurate in your preparation efforts. Here is an example of a task list for a family holiday gathering:

FAMILY HOLIDAY GATHERING

Put on nice clothes.
Get backpack (already packed).
Get in car.
Play with toys (from backpack).
Get out of car.
Walk into Grandma's house.
Say "hi" to Grandma.
Say "hi" to Grandpa.
Go to basement.
Watch *SpongeBob SquarePants* DVD.
Walk with Mom to dinner.
Eat.
Wait.
Open present.
Say "thank you."
Bathroom time.
Go to kitchen table.
Play with play dough with cousins Kate and Ray.
Go to basement.

Watch *Spider-Man* DVD.

Say "good-bye" to Grandma.

Say "good-bye" to Grandpa.

This task list gives the child with autism a clear sequence of activities to do during the unstructured periods. Remember, task lists are to be listed according to the child's eye view while the knowledge of the general format is for your understanding of the overall picture of the event. Look carefully at your list, and consider carefully whether your child can follow this particular sequence of events.

Once these tasks are listed, it is time to mark each step as one your child can do independently (**I**) or one that will need to be prompted (**P**). Maybe after writing this task list, you've realized your child doesn't use the words "thank you" upon receiving items—but you feel your child could definitely do it if taught. Possibly you could model the behavior behind the scenes, and practice at home, so your child will be able to spontaneously, or with a partial verbal prompt, say "thank you" upon receiving a gift.

Next, you need to evaluate your expectations, so that you can make a sound judgment on the duration of your stay or your child's level of involvement. Will your child be able to greet others in the excitement and commotion? Will your child have a meltdown if unexpectedly hugged?

Let's say that the initial entering and greeting period may truly be an issue for your child because of some tactile defensiveness. In your preparation, it may be a good idea to write a family letter to those who will be at the event. In this letter, you can include some general family news, but also include the important information about your child with autism that they should know. For instance, you should include the best way to communicate with your child, or the fact that your child does not like to be touched. This information will be greatly appreciated because no one attending the event would want to make your child with special issues feel uncomfortable or upset. This is a win-win step that could make the experience smoother for everyone.

After evaluating your expectations, you will need to scrutinize the environment the gathering will be held in, and determine whether accommodations need to be put in place so your child will be at his or her best. Maybe you feel you will need to designate a bedroom as a break area or quiet area, in case your child gets "overstimulated." Perhaps you feel it would benefit your child to arrive early to avoid the commotion of guests' arrivals. Your child could be safely down in the basement watching *SpongeBob SquarePants* before the holiday commotion commences. Perhaps you feel that you must kindly ask the grandparents to remove breakable items from areas your child will be in. One accommodation may be to ask a member of the family to stay with your child while you make sure to spend some quality time with your spouse and other kids.

Lastly, in preparation for the family holiday gathering, prepare a visual depiction or chart of the gathering's components from beginning to end. If your child feels stress from the novel situation, the visuals will help your child to understand where he or she is within the event, and when it will be ending.

Pre–Family Holiday Gathering Considerations

When it comes to family holiday gatherings, there are some unique aspects to consider. One of these is the special clothing that children are given to wear. Even if your child is fine initially with the feel of the more dressy clothing items, it may be a good idea to keep a change of clothes with you or in your car. If a child with autism becomes overheated or cold, or physically uncomfortable, he or she may begin to feel the "feeling" of the different clothing more. So keep favorite clothing items nearby just in case.

Also, gifts can be an issue with children with autism, because they can be very picky about what they like and don't like. For those kids that are verbal, some inappropriate comments may be made upon opening certain gifts. You can cue your child to say "thank you" or practice opening wrapped objects at home— where your child would be prompted to say "thank you" no matter the object.

Eating may also become an issue if your child is used to eating at certain times, and the serving time of food at the gathering may be different than the typical norm for your child. This can be handled by speaking with the hostess or by bringing food with you. You can have your child sit down for "lunch" or "dinner" even if the amount is snack size. The off setting of when your child typically eats can affect more than toileting. It can affect their sleep, their moods, their taking of meds, and more.

Also, always try to have a "bag of tricks" with you that contains some preferred objects, sensory toys, and some favorite snacks.

Post–Family Holiday Gathering Debriefings

After each holiday gathering your family attends, take a minute and ask yourself the following questions:

1. What successes did my child experience at the holiday gathering?

2. Was the event enjoyed by my child?

3. Was I, myself, able to socialize with family? Is there someone I could ask or bring for additional help next time?

4. Was there a particular extended family member my child was comfortable with and could perhaps spend more time with outside of holiday events?

5. Am I happy with my choice of introduction for the family gathering?

6. Was I able to accurately determine the tasks involved?

7. Were my expectations appropriate?

8. Do I want to make note of areas to accommodate better next time?

9. Did my child attend to the visuals I supplied?

With each family holiday gathering you attend with your child, you will keep making important distinctions about how to help your child to self-regulate in novel situations. With repeated exposure to family members and holiday gatherings, the familiarity of what occurs at gatherings such as these will help your child's comfort level to grow. And this in turn will bring about increased interactions and communicative behaviors within these gatherings.

Let's take a look at the experiences other moms of autistic kids have had at holiday times.

Examples of Family Holiday Gatherings and the Value of I.D.E.A.L.

In the past several years, we have only gone to a couple family dinners or get-togethers—which were both disasters, so I would either hold an easy family party, like a Halloween thing, or Valentine's party, or just skip festivities with Dante all together. He would open presents on Christmas, but it has always been in our house with just us. Before Dante, I had pretty elaborate Christmas parties, so I decided to throw one of my long lost Christmas parties—even so my daughter could experience it for the first time. My husband, daughter, and I went through the steps of I.D.E.A.L. together, and we found it exciting to do because it even helped us to plan and envision our party as we went. We used Google to find pictures on the computer and made Dante a "social story" to introduce what would happen, we chose a reasonable format together, and my daughter was just key in helping to list the tasks from Dante's eyes. Dante would need a lot of escapes and a lot of breaks, so we planned to put a portable DVD player in Dante's bedroom on the evening of the party. My daughter thought of the idea of putting a couple containers of snacks in his room on that night, too. I know some parents have high expectations for their kids with autism, and that they would want them to be involved in some way in every activity, but for me, I just wanted him to be all right in the presence of a party going on. If he needed to be alone for a while, that would be fine with me. My daughter would keep him company if he retreated to his room, or my husband and I would take turns checking on him. I did end up including a form letter in the invitations that told everyone about Dante, and his difficulties with communication and noise.

I made a visual schedule for him by taking pictures of my daughter doing different activities, because I couldn't get Dante himself to sit for the pictures.

Well, this experience ended up being very interesting, because in the preparation for the party, we discovered that Dante has an interest in cooking! He actually helped make some of the Christmas cookies! He also acted differently at the actual Christmas party than we expected. Instead of retreating to his room—which I expected him to do—he sat for a long, long time on the stairwell watching everyone and holding his activity chart. It was as if he was watching the activities on the chart go by in real life. It was a big learning moment for my husband and I to see that this "real life" event was more interesting to him than the movies in his room. It was a surprise to us, and still is when I think about it. The experience was food for thought. I would highly recommend I.D.E.A.L.

My sister was holding a Passover seder at her house, and we decided to go this year as an entire family. Usually I would go, and my husband would stay with Jared at home. I wrote a "social story" and bought a picture book too to introduce Jared to what would be happening. A seder is like a religious service and dinner combined, so I knew Jared would not be able to sit through it, and when I did the task list part of I.D.E.A.L., it just seemed like way too much to ask of poor Jared. So, I spoke with my sister, and we decided to shorten the duration, and arrive at the eating portion of the seder. I thought this would work well because there is a kids' time soon after eating where afikomen, a special piece of mat-zoh, is hidden and the kids have to try to find it. My sister's son was going to try to get Jared to look with him around the house. This seemed to enthuse Jared when we read the "social story," and I knew it would give him a time where it was perfectly okay to move around. Jared's activity schedule only had a few things on it, but he did look at it, and used it while we were there. I think my plan for a shortened seder worked really well for us. We arrived late and left early, but we went as a family, and got to visit with our family. The planning helped us make some good choices for Jared.

My mother-in-law throws a cute Easter party and egg hunt for the grandchildren, and my two older ones have always gone and enjoyed themselves, so I decided to bring Caleb this year. My mother-in-law was not so sure she was ready to handle Caleb around the others, so I let her know we would be doing some special planning and told her not to worry. Caleb bites, and he has bitten my mother-in-law a couple times, so she acts, and feels, I guess, tentative around him. I asked my mother-in-law if I could take pictures of her, her house, and her backyard, and I made a photographic walk book for Caleb with those pictures and pictures I cut out from magazines—like colored eggs, and baskets—things like that. Because he bites when he gets agitated, I bought fruit snacks and Easter marshmallows to accommodate his oral needs, and bought enough in case some of the other kids would want some, too. One of the issues that came up for me was the Easter egg hunt in the back yard. Her yard is not fenced, and I didn't know if I would be able to con-tain Caleb in that one area. I had mentioned this to my mother-in-law, and lo and behold, she got volunteers from her church to come to the party and stand in various places along the perimeter. She solved it for me! Caleb seemed to know exactly what to do when we got there. He wanted his basket and to get on with his search. He ate a lot of marshmallows, but bit no one, and found five eggs on his own. At one point he went to stand like some of the men he saw along the perimeter, and stood on guard for a while. I.D.E.A.L. was a nice tool to use. And it's also easy to remember.

CHAPTER 14

■   ■   ■

Recreational Activities

Our coach put a big cardboard Barney picture on the goal post so Drew would know which way to run with the ball. At first, we all thought it was kind of embarrassing 'cause it was Barney, but now if you make a goal, you get to sign your name on Barney, and everyone wants to make a goal and do it.

—*VINCE*, age ten,
friend and team member of Drew, who has autism

For all children, familiarity can bring about comfort with other kids, and over time recreational activities are the perfect conduits to establishing this ease. Repeated exposure to a specific group of peers gives children with autism ample time and chances to find a true companion and friend, as well as the time needed to display some of their strengths. Repeated exposure to a group also allows for an autistic child's communication style to be observed and learned. Once the mystery of how to communicate with the autistic child has been discovered by peers, the willingness of all the children to interact and form bonds increases.

Recreational activity possibilities can support and highlight your child's interests and strengths, so look back at the choices of activities you noted in Chapter Five, and think about the steps of I.D.E.A.L. and how using the steps will help your child get involved. By previewing and planning recreational activities using the I.D.E.A.L. system, we will look at the special considerations that will need to be addressed, such as making any needed accommodations, initiating conversations with coaches, combing recreation sites for safety issues, and introducing new skills and tasks.

All the knowledge you have learned thus far will benefit your child in recreational settings. If needed, your child can use a schedule of reinforcement, or take sensory breaks during an activity. Your child will be able to attend for the amount of time that is right for her, and your child will "know the drill" from her visual schedule.

Your preparation and efforts to prime your child will pay off. The reward of witnessing your child interact and try new skills in social recreational settings will be priceless.

The Sequential Steps of a Recreational Activity

Recreational activities differ from playdates and parties in that they often require a period of listening to directions, and a possible rapid gathering of materials. Some recreational activities meet in one environment, but then quickly move to another. These are details that can and should be found out beforehand. In sports and recreation, there is usually no repetition of directions once they are given, so children with autism, including higher-functioning kids, often need some accommodations in this area. Visual activity charts help enormously when kids' have weak language processing.

Let's take a look at some example formats for recreational activities:

FORMAT A

Initial entering experience
Greeting
Listening to directions
Sustained group activity
Good-bye

FORMAT B

Initial entering experience
Greeting
Listening to directions
Gathering of materials
Sustained individual activity
Putting away of materials
Good-bye

FORMAT C

Initial entering experience
Greeting
Listening to directions
Gathering of materials
Transition of location
Sustained group activity 1

Break
Sustained group activity 2
Transition of location
Putting away of materials
Good-bye

FORMAT D

Initial entering experience
Greeting
Listening to directions
Sustained individual activity 1
Sustained group activity 2
Listening to directions
Good-bye

You may have noticed the different language in these formats, such as, *sustained group activity* and *sustained individual activity*. A sustained group activity is one that requires a sustained awareness and reciprocity with others, such as a game of soccer or tag. A sustained individual activity requires sustained individual focus (and not interaction) to complete the activity, such as an arts and crafts activity or swimming. There is a difference in the stamina and attention required in these activities, so again, refer to your child's strengths, and choose an activity and format that may work well for him.

Transitioning from one location to another can also pose a challenge for children with autism, and transitioning is a common step in many recreational activities. Kids move from locker rooms to playing fields or pools, and from classrooms to outdoor areas, so kids with autism will often need to be accommodated with special plans. Sometimes, very simple techniques do the trick for kids, such as getting several prewarnings before the move to a different location, or seeing the next location on a visual activity chart. Some children enjoy using active patterns (see Chapter Three) when transitioning from one location to another.

When you go through the steps of I.D.E.A.L., you will be able to consider the parts of an activity your child will be able to handle independently and the parts that will need to be assisted. Let's look at an example of planning for a recreational activity including some of the new issues that will need to be addressed, such as direction following and transitioning in recreational settings.

Previewing and Planning a Recreational Activity Using I.D.E.A.L.

- **I**ntroduce the Activity.

- **D**etermine the Tasks Involved.

- **E**valuate Your Expectations.

- **A**ccommodate for Success.

- **L**ist the Activity Components Visually.

As with all of our social outings thus far, you will first need to choose your mode of introducing the recreational activity to your child, and for recreational activities, there are many supplementary options to use in introducing both sports as well as artistic pursuits. If you choose a "social story" or photographic walk of the actual venue and instructors, don't hesitate to also show your child video clips from Internet sites, and books from the library or bookstore that have interesting visuals, or text (if your child reads) about the activity your child will be participating in. Stop your car alongside a soccer field and sit and watch the players run across the field while kicking the ball. There are many possibilities you can turn to, to help your child learn what to expect and what will be expected during recreational activities.

After introducing the activity to your child, you will want to determine the tasks involved as accurately as you can. Call the recreation facility and ask to speak with one of the staff members who will be running your child's program. Let the person know that, to prepare your child, you will need to know the general order of activities. If the information you are given is very brief, you may have to ask some good questions to find out exactly when the directions are given, or when a break is given, and whether the children will have to move from one location to another during the duration of the activity. As you are given the sequence of events, write them down so you can clearly see the general format. Then write out a task list of sequential steps your child would have to complete from beginning to end in order to successfully participate in the activity. Let's use joining a karate class as an example activity to analyze. Here's what your child might have to do:

KARATE CLASS

Get in karate uniform.
Get in car.
Get out of car.
Walk with Dad into building.
Find karate room.
Say (possibly bow) hello to teacher.
Run.

Do push-ups.

Go stand in place.

Do karate moves.

Go with partner.

Do karate moves with partner.

Go stand in place.

Say (possibly bow) good-bye to teacher.

Walk with Dad to car.

Get into car.

Get out of car.

Walk with Dad into house.

Take off karate uniform.

This task list looks doable, and would be pretty simple to make into a visual chart for your child to follow.

But let's say in the next step—evaluating your expectations— several issues come up from your knowledge of your child. Let's say you are worried about two things: your child being able to stand in one spot during the class, even with the other kids modeling the correct behavior, and also the pairing of kids to practice movements. Possibly you are worried your child will hurt someone by not being able to appropriately grade his or her movements, or may forcefully hit a peer. Though you feel your child could handle the duration of the class, which is one hour, you know that in the next step of I.D.E.A.L., these issues would need to be accommodated. After marking each step with the letters **I** or **P** (**I**: your child can do the step independently, or **P**: your child will need to be prompted), you can get to work on accommodating for success. For the concerns noted from the task list, possibly your child can be given a visual marker to stand on that is just for him. An X made from colored tape or a big smiley face taped to the floor can mark the spot your child needs to go to each time the kids are expected to stand in a line or in rows. This would be an easy personal accommodation that would not affect the other class members at all (unless they all want one, too).

To accommodate the worries about inappropriate force when kids are paired to spar with each other, possibly you can ask the teacher if your child can spar with him, instead of another peer. The teacher may or may not go for this. They may feel they would not be able to instruct or advise the rest of the class. One other accommodation is to have your child initially exit before the sparring section of the activity, and model and practice sparring at home until you have some confidence your child is able to grade his or her movements. You may be able to have the instructor give your child a couple private tutoring sessions on sparring in pairs.

After going through the steps of I.D.E.A.L., and weighing some careful considerations, your child's task list may look like this:

KARATE CLASS

Get in karate uniform.
Get in car.
Get out of car.
Walk with Dad into building.
Find karate room.
Say (possibly bow) hello to teacher.
Run.
Do push-ups.
Go stand in place.
Do karate moves.
Say (possibly bow) good-bye to teacher.

Walk with Dad to car.

Get into car.

Get out of car.

Walk with Dad into house.

Take off karate uniform.

Lastly, preparing a visual chart with pictures, text, or both, will help your child keep track of what comes next, and the components of the recreational activity. It will help your child clearly understand the beginning, middle, and end of what he or she is doing.

Pre–Recreational Activity Considerations

Recreational activities are numerous and varied, but as you prepare to sign your child up, one common issue that must be addressed will be how much information needs to be given to staff members on your child's diagnosis and skills—and when. A lot of parents are hesitant to be completely forthcoming about their kids' behaviors and deficits for fear of discrimination—from staff, or from parents of other kids signed up. There is also a little something about always having to "give the autism info" again and again that makes parents feel as if they're making their child sound like a clinical disease rather than a loving individual. And it's frustrating when you feel that.

Recreational staff I have spoken with over the years have mentioned that when they find out one of the participants has autism and that's all they're told—they have no idea what the child will be like or what they would need to do or not do. They become extremely frustrated when there is "no information attached," and they worry whether they will be able to handle a child with autism while handling the other children at the same time.

I would recommend that you be honest at the time of sign-up, and provide a simple information sheet about your child that can be attached to the registration form. Be accurate about skills and behaviors, but be brief. At the bottom of the information sheet include a note that says you welcome phone calls, and include your phone number. You can photocopy this information sheet and use it throughout a six-month period or year (if it still applies) for activities, doctor's appointments, and even religious classes.

Here's what your information sheet should include:

Child's name:
Child's age and grade:
Child's diagnosis:
Child's communication system:
Child's general likes/strengths:
Child's general dislikes/weaknesses:
Behaviors that may need to be addressed:
Triggers for those behaviors:
Best ways to handle behaviors:
Attending with an adult to assist? Yes or No (circle one)
Feel free to call me, _____
        at (#) _____.

Depending on the type of recreational activity your child gets involved in, some staff may ask to see your child's IEP.

I would also like to mention that you need to use care and common sense when choosing recreational activities for your child. I used karate as an example of an activity but I would not recommend it for several of the kids I have worked with. You will have to consider your child's level of judgment. For instance, you do not want your child using their newly learned karate moves on children on the playground, or on their teachers at school. You really need to think about how learning to use certain movements, tools, or sports equipment will benefit your child. Does your child have the reasoning skills and judgment to use the tools and lessons appropriately? There are many choices for activities. Choose wisely.

Post–Recreational Activity Debriefings

After each recreational experience your child has, take a few moments and ask yourself the following questions:

1. What successes did my child experience at the recreational activity?

2. Was the activity enjoyed by my child?

3. Did my child connect with a peer I would want to pursue for friendship for my child?

4. Am I happy with my choice of recreational facility?

5. Was I able to accurately determine the tasks involved?

6. Were my expectations appropriate?

7. Do I want to make note of areas to accommodate better next time?

8. Did my child attend to the visuals I supplied?

As children with autism gain familiarity with the people and expectations within a recreational activity, they can really progress with the activity skills and begin to interact much more with their peers. Do not feel uncomfortable about experimenting with different durations or accommodations. You can slowly work toward longer durations, and once you get out there more with your child, you will know from experience exactly what accommodations really make the difference.

Take a look at the experiences of other moms when planning for and involving their children with autism in recreational activities.

Examples of Recreational Activities and the Value of I.D.E.A.L.

My son, Eric, I am happy to say, is a tennis player now, like his father and I. We decided to try tennis with I.D.E.A.L. and originally my first concern was the racket. I didn't really expect at first for this to work out well, so I bought a really cheap little used racket, which I have since replaced. I was scared my son would hit someone or himself with the racket because he does do some self-injurious scratching when he gets agitated.

I introduced the activity by giving him a photographic walk of our community center, and I brought him to see my husband and I play tennis, but he only wanted to sit in the car. I called to meet the tennis instructor, who was a little nervous about Eric, but up for the challenge, and I promised him that my husband or I would always be there assisting Eric.

I determined the tasks involved and then felt like I had

chosen the wrong activity, because I didn't think Eric would even see the ball coming. But my husband sat with me and we started talking about accommodations, and then we came up with some ideas we really thought would work. We decided to accommodate Eric by not reducing the duration of the activity, but by extending the duration. We decided to bring Eric early, and let him walk around the outskirts of the courts a little, and then we would use little blow-up beach balls for him to hit in the class, at least in the beginning. The beach balls were bright colors and large in comparison to the tennis balls, but we later replaced them with orange tennis balls once he got the hang of hitting a ball.

Eric isn't able to play a tennis game yet, but you can throw a ball and he will swing and hit it. Kids in the tennis class will throw balls to him when it is not their turn on the court. We used a visual schedule with Eric and did put a token system along the bottom where he swings and tries to hit five times, and then sits down on the side for five minutes of holding a vibrating ladybug toy. His improvement with hitting balls is spectacular, and we never would have come up with our beach ball idea if it weren't for taking a minute to brainstorm accommodations. We have continued with tennis for Eric, and he seems to love it.

Our daughter, Sasha, has autism and she has always been attracted to music. When we were going through a list of activities, and trying to really highlight her strengths, an activity like dancing really caught our attention. When I introduced the activity to her with a "social story," I couldn't tell if she was interested or not, so I added some pictures from the Web to the "social story," and that really piqued her interest.

I had a couple different options for dance classes in our community and chose one that I thought would work well because there would be less kids, and the teacher was just really open to Sasha's joining. I then made a photographic walk for Sasha of the actual dance room, teacher, and took a picture of an older group during a class. When I determined the tasks involved and thought about my expectations, I felt unsure of what I was writing, so I called the dance teacher, and spoke more in depth with her about what would be happening and this made all the difference for my list of tasks and making sure Sasha would have a visual chart that was true to the class's activities.

The dance teacher was willing to try to prompt Sasha so that I would not have to, and she was able to do this at least some of the time. Sasha has come to love her dance class, and she watches and tries to do what the other children are doing with their bodies as best she can. She now wants to see on our calendar at home if the day is a "dance day." Many of the other girls like to help Sasha and will buddy up with her, and one girl just recently gave her a birthday invitation, so back to I.D.E.A.L. once more!

Our son is physically affected, nonverbal, and very sensitive, but he has always shown an interest in his older brother's soccer. Benny would excitedly pace and flap along the edge of the field and around our chairs, but he has always been afraid of going on the field past that boundary line. I chose to sign him up for soccer. Our community knows Benny, and a few neighbors thought I was crazy, but it is what he loves and enjoys.

To my understanding with I.D.E.A.L., I could determine tasks for my son according to my well-considered expectations, and what I want and expect for him is to find a way to be involved in what he loves. I do not expect him to be a typical team member, but I expect others to make allowances for my son so he can be involved in some way, and I will happily bring him for ten minutes to do something small for or with the team if it makes him happy.

As we were putting together a photographic walk for Benny, my older son approached me and said, "Ben can throw the ball in." I had to kiss him when he said that. We went with that, I left a message for the coach, and the coach agreed to give Benny that job. And he loves it. It has also become such a mission for some of the kids on the soccer team to teach Benny how to kick a ball, that I was asked by one of the kids to add a picture of "kick" onto Benny's visual schedule.

CHAPTER 15

■   ■   ■

Family Restaurant Visits and Trips

It bothered me a lot when I was younger 'cause we'd be out, and people would look at us and stuff, and some people would move to different seats. I try to say to myself, "That's a person that doesn't know about autism," but it can get you angry sometimes. It's not like he can help it . . . that he has autism.

—ROBERT, *age eleven,*
big brother to James, who has autism

Eating out and traveling pose some unique challenges for children with autism and their families. Often this is due to behaviors caused by sensory sensitivities, changes to the child's typical daily routines, and the unwelcome looks, comments, and contact with insensitive strangers. Many moms of autistic children I work with mention the discomfort and even anger they feel in reaction to "looks" and thoughtless comments from those on the outside looking in. As a result of their experiences, many of them simply stop going out.

It is hard to cope with "stranger intrusions" while simultaneously trying to remain focused on your family members and "family time." There will be moments you want to take people by the shoulders and let them know loudly and clearly that you are ignoring your child because it is part of his behavior plan. Children with autism are no doubt going to have their "moments" out in public, and they may be embarrassing, but we need to remind ourselves that these moments are what they are: overload poor judgment on their part, or our part, the kids' emerging awareness, attempts at getting attention, asserting oneself, or socializing inappropriately. Our children need to learn to cope among real people in the real world.

Here are two ways to deal with stranger intrusions:

- Try to exude warmth, through your facial expressions and body language. Your calm handling of any behaviors can tip strangers" attitudes in your favor. Simple phrases, such as "Excuse us" or "My son has autism and is a little overwhelmed," paired with a warm, friendly facial expression, can truly take strangers from being hurtful to helpful.

- Have a few pamphlets or preprinted cards handy that may provide information as simple as, "This is a child with Autism, for more information contact . . . [website]." It may do the trick when your hands are full.

When you have a plan in mind about how you will be handling the strangers on the outside looking in and decide to take the high road in the situation, you will find that instead of feeling embarrassed by ignorant remarks, you will feel empowered to kindly educate others. Change comes from new knowledge, and you may end up helping a great many people you encounter on your outings and in your travels to change their views.

Unfortunately, traveling and eating in restaurants are often strictly avoided by families that have children with autism, so let's take a look at some of the steps involved with going out and with travel, so we can get you and your family out to dinner and on your way to some great destinations.

The Sequential Steps of a Special Outing

Going to restaurants can be challenging for children with autism because there is an unknown amount of open-ended waiting, as well as aromas, sounds, and visual effects that may not agree with the child. It can be helpful to plan to go to a more family-oriented restaurant where your child may not be noticed above and beyond the movement and noises of other people's kids. But again, with preplanning, it is possible to work out accommodations that will suit your child's needs and allow you to revisit some of your favorite dinner spots.

With traveling, the many issues to consider can be overwhelming, so it is best to begin with one single question:

What does my child absolutely need to have every day?

As you answer this question, you will begin to have a list that may include such things as medications, special diet foods, preferred objects, and preferred books or DVDs. What you will notice is that you do not have to bring your child's bed—maybe just a favorite blanket or pillow, and you do not have to bring your child's entire DVD library—maybe just five really key films.

You want to have the important preferred and familiar items with you. When you are traveling, make a format you can refer to, and give each piece some special consideration.

Let's take a look at a sample format for a restaurant outing and a sample format for a trip departure:

RESTAURANT OUTING FORMAT

Initial entering experience
Walk through to table
Wait time 1
Ordering
Wait time 2
Eating
Wait time 3
Walk through to door

TRIP DEPARTURE FORMAT

Car travel
Initial entering experience
Airport walk-through
Wait time 1
Board plane
Initial entering experience
Plane walk-through
Wait time 2
Takeoff experience
Open-ended flight time
Landing experience
Disembark plane
Initial entering experience

Airport walk-through
Gather luggage (Wait time 3)
Exit

What these outings have in common are extensive wait times or multiple amounts of time that need to be structured and filled. Waiting is difficult and uncomfortable for kids with autism, and kids will find ways to fill the time—for instance, they may start self-stimming or they may begin to engage in inappropriate behavior. It is important to help the children have ways to appropriately spend their wait times.

When you are going on any special outing with your child, you should bring some preferred objects and activities, and bring enough of them so that you can cover the time. And I am not talking about packing boxes of toys. Kids with autism also love little things like rubber bands, tape, calculators, mini electronic games, flip books, and tiny plastic animals—and a lot of little objects can keep the children busy.

Kids may also need special preferred items to distract them from uncomfortable sensory sensations, which can include anything from dimmed lighting in restaurants to loudspeakers and plane engine noise at airports. Headphones, CD players, and iPods can all help to distract kids who are sensitive to their environments.

Previewing and Planning Special Outings Using I.D.E.A.L.

- **I**ntroduce the Activity.

- **D**etermine the Tasks Involved.

- **E**valuate Your Expectations.

- **A**ccommodate for Success.

- **L**ist the Activity Components Visually.

To prime your child for a special outing, you will need to introduce the activity, just as you have with playdates, parties, and recreational activities. If you are using photographs for a restaurant outing, try to get pictures of the restaurant at a similar time of day to when you will be going. For instance, if you will be going at night when it will be dark, try to take pictures of what the restaurant looks like inside and out when it's dark. If you are preparing an introduction about a trip, get photos from online sites about your hotels and destination attractions. This will help familiarize your child with what is to come. I like for parents to add little touches to motivate their child, such as including in their "social story" or photographic walk that a favorite movie will be in the hotel room, or that a favorite toy will sit with the child on the plane.

When it is time to determine the tasks involved, this is obviously easier to do for a two- to three-hour dinner than a five-day trip. When you are traveling, it is a good idea to focus on one day at a time, and prepare for just one day at a time. You may need to recycle some DVDs and preferred objects, but this usually is fine with the kids. Sometimes you will see your child attracted to little souvenirs that can be bought and used as time fillers or rewards. You may want to find out if certain markets or stores are in your destination's area beforehand.

We will use a restaurant outing as an example for our task list and to determine the tasks involved. Possibly it will be an anniversary dinner, or a celebration dinner of some kind.

Remember, we write our task list steps from looking at the activity components from the child's eye view.

RESTAURANT OUTING

Get in car.
Look at book.
Get out of car.
Walk with Mom and Dad into restaurant.
Follow Mom and Dad to table.
Sit down.
Look at menu.
Wait.
Say, "I want pizza."
Play with calculator.
Eat pizza.
Play with toy animals.
Say, "I want fruit."
Play with animals.
Wipe hands and face.
Walk with Mom and Dad to door.
Get in car.

While determining the tasks involved, you may have already prepared for many of the wait times you observed in the basic format of what your child would experience at the restaurant. You can see from the task list that you have already planned to bring your bag of tricks with you, including a calculator and toy or cut-out animals. You may have noticed I included that your child looks at the menu, and uses some "I want" phrases. It is sometimes fun to make a menu of items your child recognizes and can say, and just bring it, or if you visit the restaurant before-hand, you can borrow one of their menus, and you can tape in a menu you make from pictures you get on the Internet—so your child will feel like she is holding a similar menu to yours (on the outside at least). If possible, prompt your child to use some language or gestures for something she wants.

When you are evaluating your expectations for an outing like this restaurant visit, you need to determine the duration you feel your child can handle. Waiting is really a huge issue, so you may want to speak with the restaurant staff and find out how much time it generally takes to be served there. Possibly going at an earlier hour may reduce the wait time, or ask if you can order your food by phone before leaving your house. The food could be brought out soon after you are seated, and this would shorten the duration of the experience if needed, for your child.

If you plan ahead and call in advance, accommodations will often be honored by restaurant staff, so if you feel your family will need special seating, for instance, such as a table close to the restrooms or close to (or away from) a door, most restaurants will try to accommodate you.

Some families like to bring a helper with them to dinner—especially when the dinner has special significance. Helpers may be paraprofessionals from your child's school, recreational staff, or even neighborhood babysitters, or family members willing to help out. A helper can take your child for a walk if she is getting antsy, or take your child to the car to watch a part of a movie, or to play a game that would be inappropriate to play in the restaurant.

As with the previous social activities and events, you will want your child to have a visual task list with pictures, words, or both, so she will know what will be happening.

Pre–Special Outing Considerations

An important consideration for outings and travel with autistic kids is how very hard it is for them to navigate unstructured "free" time. Though downtime may seem like a period of relaxation to us, the openness of time can cause children with autism to feel a lot of stress that manifests as self-stimulation behaviors, disengaging behaviors, and irritability. Keeping kids happy means keeping kids busy on outings. This does not mean that kids have to be kept busy with action-packed days. A lot of activities can be quieter activities or calming sensory tasks. The ebb and flow on trips should be similar to the pattern of your days at home, meaning that you eat breakfast, lunch, and dinner at similar times to your routine at home. And if your child naps at a certain time or goes to sleep at a certain time, try to keep these times as similar as possible to your patterns at home.

On outings and on trips, expect that your child will need many preferred objects and activities, and that he will need several breaks for snacks, sensory input, or simply quiet. Some families like to bring two cars on trips just in case one parent may need to run back to the hotel with their autistic child. This way they can leave and rejoin as needed without disturbing the experience for all of the family members.

When traveling, you also may want to call ahead to your airline, train, or bus company to discuss seating. If your child may disturb others by playing with a tray attached to the seat in front, or disturb others by kicking the seat in front, request special seating, either in the first row, or plan to have a family member sit directly in the seat in front of your child with autism.

Also, several destinations have special accommodations for

disabled children and adults. Many families with children with autism have been thrilled with the *special assistance passes* that parks like Disneyland and Disney World give out. The passes help to cut out standing and waiting time and offer special accommodations that make the park easier to access.

Post–Special Outing Debriefings

After each special outing or travel experience with your child, take a couple minutes and ask yourself the following questions:

1. What successes did my child experience on the outing/trip?

2. What was enjoyed by my child?

3. Which part(s) of the outing/trip was the hardest for my child?

4. Am I happy with my choice of place/destination?

5. Would I change the duration of time spent at this place/destination?

6. Were my expectations appropriate?

7. Do I want to make note of areas to accommodate better next time?

8. Did my child attend to the visuals I supplied?

Preplanning and preparation are extremely important when you are going on an outing or a trip. With that said, kids with autism do often make it through outings and trips like troupers. It can be an adventure with high highs and low lows, but if you really look carefully at the issues you will face, the experience will *not* overwhelm you, or your child.

Here are some examples of how other moms planned for outings and traveled with their children with autism.

Examples of Outings and the Value of I.D.E.A.L.

We took our family to Mystic and Mystic Aquarium and our son loved it. We made him a book of pictures to introduce our trip to him, and it was a real motivator. I made him task lists for the trip which ended up being his daily visual itinerary schedules, and we called ahead to both the hotel and aquarium to find out what was available to us as far as accommodations for the disabled. Our hotel allowed us to check in at an earlier time, and we reserved a room on the ground floor because Dominic likes to run and jump.

I brought a duffel bag full of his preferred movies, books, and toys, and he enjoyed rummaging through the bag both days we were there. We stayed only overnight, but it was an experiment for us—a successful one, so I would like to go for two nights next time. Our hotel room had a fridge in it, so I kept Dom's favorite drinks, snacks, and breakfast foods accessible at all times. While we were at the aquarium, Dom did start to melt down at one point, and I asked one of the people that worked there if there was a quiet spot nearby, and he immediately helped me lead Dom to a classroom-style room that was not being used. I quietly sang a couple of Dom's favorite songs, and then asked if he wanted to see the sea lions, and we were off again. I feel the planning worked very well, and I thank you for putting the pieces of I.D.E.A.L. together.

We took a beach trip and it had been many years since we last took a vacation like this. I think we just never knew what to expect traveling with a child with autism. When we started really looking at doing this, and doing the steps for planning ahead of time, we decided to be smart and not go during the typical tourist times like the summer months. The car ride would be about four hours, so we decided to stop every hour for one reason or another.

And I brought lots of things for Jake to do. And I tried to follow each step of I.D.E.A.L. as best I could. I even made him some character rule lists for play at the ocean and when in the hotel room. I had introduced the trip to Jake with a "social story"—the first one I ever wrote—and he took to it well. I listed tasks we were doing for each day and did the write-on wipe board, which I had with me at all times, even on the beach. I liked it because it worked for Jake, and I could constantly erase and revise it. Someone on the beach saw me using it and asked if Jake was deaf—just thought I'd throw that in there.

I think Jake surpassed my expectations. He played longer on the beach and in the pool than I expected. And he went to sleep in the hotel bed—I guess out of exhaustion. But I hadn't expected him to fall off to sleep like he did.

We went to Washington, D.C., this past spring because we have family there (this was our personal accommodation), and there is a wonderful zoo and museums that I knew our kids would love. Ashley is my typical child, and Derek is my autistic child, and Derek probably loved the Air and Space Museum more than anything else. So much so, that we had to go there repeatedly—but none of us minded. We took the train down, and the kids played with their Nintendos and snacked most of the way.

I made an elaborate introduction poster for Derek that was hung in his room for the entire week before going. We brought this poster on the train with us, and safety-pinned it to the seatbacks in front of the kids so Derek wouldn't touch those trays! We went over the story several times with him on the train. I also made him an activity schedule, that I will make a smaller version of next time, but it worked.

We don't have to worry about too many behaviors with Derek, but he gets very anxious, so the pictures helped him. And I will continue to use visuals more with him because I did feel they made a difference. We bought Derek several little souvenirs and a couple books from the Air and Space Museum and he just devoured those books and the pamphlets on the train ride back. We accommodated by pinning a towel to the seatbacks on the way back.

CONCLUSION

A socially included child will be a more successful child. Each and every outing and new social experience will give your child the practice and the familiarity needed to learn to cope with and function within the different work and leisure environments he or she may need to move through more independently as a teen or an adult. Your child will gain the pertinent social experience needed for dealing with different types of people in various types of environments.

A knowledgeable parent will be a well-prepared parent. The experience of socially including your child as a young person will enable you to help your son or daughter by pulling from and reusing known and successful strategies that circumvent the weaknesses and discomforts that make him or her struggle. Your son or daughter will be able to interact more comfortably, with the confidence built from experience and personal accomplishments.

A Child's Social Future

Though we are advised by some not to do this, most of us find ourselves looking into the future trying to imagine our kids five or ten years down the road—wondering where they will be with their skills and behaviors, and what adulthood might look like for them. Common questions are, "Will my child be able to hold a job and live independently?" and, "Will my child have a group of true friends that he or she can trust?" Children with autism can and do continue to learn new skills as they move into their teen years and young adulthood, and the journey to job success and satisfaction will be different for each individual. It is always helpful for children with autism, as they grow into young adults, to have family and friends they can rely upon to freely give them ongoing lessons and guidance, so that they can make appropriate adjustments, if necessary, in behavior or in their choices, or even in their self-care.

I.D.E.A.L. is an important tool, and some children, as they grow older, will be able to take on the routine action steps of I.D.E.A.L. and plan or perform some of the steps independently, or offer input to help advocate for themselves. I.D.E.A.L. helps children to function in natural social environments that, unfortunately, for the young people with autism, include elements of surprise, and unplanned interactions that can make them uncomfortable. But the kids will be able to lean on their prior experiences with I.D.E.A.L. and their social inclusion, and their experiences with previewing. Young people with autism will put to good use the experimentation with and use of the simple accommodations that worked well for them. Experience and lots of practice do make a difference for children with autism.

Core Interests

As you socially include your child, you will begin to notice that some interests ebb and wane, while others really stick. Many times, the activities and interests that truly attract your child over time coincide with their true strengths. As you watch your child enjoy her leisure time, make a note of the types of activities she engages in that do show her true talents. You can introduce real-life work-related elements such as numbers, schedules, paper shredding, ordering, technology, reading, stacking, drawing, et cetera, that can be used as fun and stimulating introductions to skills used within the workforce.

It may be helpful to give your child a special job within your own house to help her gain experience, independence, and self-confidence. One mother, just the other day, told me she has made her son their "recycling manager." This little boy uses a visual chart to perform the steps of his gathering and separating "job," but does it proudly and well.

We Are Independent and Interdependent

None of us are successful completely alone—independent of others. As a community and society, we are interdependent. We work with and assist one another—we all play a role in each other's daily living. And we need to teach our children with autism to work not only toward independence with their skills, but also toward interdependence with other people.

The experience of social inclusion helps children with autism learn about the interdependence that will benefit them and help them make social distinctions in approaching others, assisting others, responding, and in asking for the assistance they need—which can make their lives much more manageable on a daily basis.

A good first lesson in interdependence for younger children with autism is learning to ask for help or assistance.

Whether your child is verbal or nonverbal, he should be taught a communicative method to ask for help—even if this is handing over or pointing to a visual "help" icon or card. Toddlers can begin to be taught this lesson as soon as they begin to lead you to the food cabinet, or to a shelf with a favorite toy, or as soon as they begin to tantrum to get out of the bath or scream for a wanted item. Children with autism need to learn that people help other people. But people need to be "asked" for help.

Social Rules

The children I have worked with over the years do not pick up social intricacies the way typical peers do—some children pick up some, but the range of referencing peers and learning in social environments is vast and huge. As you know, some children just have trouble making an entrance into a social arena and are unable to attend to the models around them.

When we begin to teach social rules for appropriate behavior, we need to keep the child's developmental age or level in mind so that we can communicate at a level the child will understand. We also need to remember to describe a rule simply and literally. This means, you need to clearly state the behavior as you would "see it," without vagueness or room for interpretation. For instance, instead of saying, "You need to behave in church," you might say: "In church, you will sit with a quiet mouth, hands in your lap, and feet on the floor." As children get older, you may need to tell your child, "When you hug a friend, you may let your shoulders touch. You may not let your chest, stomach, or legs touch." I sometimes advise others to state rules as if they were on an old radio show, when scenes were described so that a clear picture could be formed in the listeners' visual minds.

Visuals can be used to help demonstrate social rules, but make sure your child understands the pictures and can correctly interpret them.

Social Self-Advocacy

When children are little, we want them to be able to assimilate with other children—join and be part of the group—run with the crowd, if you will. And many of us, as parents and teachers, give children messages that tell them: the crowd is there, and you should be, too. But as kids get older, we no longer want them to follow the crowd—for reasons involving safety and reputation. We no longer want our kids to imitate what the crowd does or how they act. And children with autism can be at risk for being easy targets for bad influence and teasing.

As you use I.D.E.A.L. in social and recreational settings, start building your child's self-confidence, so that she will feel more comfortable advocating for herself later on. Giving your child simple decisions, such as choosing which reward, snack, partner, et cetera, would be preferred, is helpful for starting your child off on beginning self-advocacy skills. You want to begin to instill in your child that she has a voice, and that her voice will be heard.

It is also beneficial to allow your child to choose her recreational activities or hobbies, and to then let her experience the results of that choice.

It is also important for your child with autism to understand that he can say "no" to another child or to an adult. Though many children early on need to learn the language and concept of "no," once understood, your child should have some practice using it. If you need to set up situations where you offer food you know your child dislikes, or offer to drive your child to an environment you know your child would avoid like the plague, do offer these options, so that your child can practice self-advocacy, and say "no." ("No, thank you" for those who are further with their language and social skills.)

As you get out more using I.D.E.A.L. and gain comfort with the process, you will notice how by simply going through each of the five key steps, a world of difference can be made for your child with autism. Remember, it is okay to start small and slowly work your way up to extended periods of time in more natural social environments. It is my hope that you will find the information that has been shared with you in this book helpful and useful. You will, no doubt, see positive results from your efforts. There is nothing like seeing your child grow and enjoy time with family and friends!

I wish all the best for you and your child.

APPENDIX

I.D.E.A.L. Resources for Social Activities

Adventure Without Limits

1341 Pacific Avenue, Forest Grove, OR 97116; (503) 359-2568

American Therapeutic Recreation Association

1414 Prince Street, Suite 204, Arlington, VA 22314; (703) 683-9420
http://atra-online.com/cms/

(The) Arc

http://www.thearc.org

(The) Arc of Multnomah County, OR

619 SW 11th Street, Portland, OR 97205; (503) 223-7279

Asperger's Syndrome Coalition of the United States

P.O. Box 9267, Jackson Beach, FL 32240; (904) 745-6741

Autism Research Institute (ATI)

http://www.autism.com

Autism Speaks

2 Park Avenue, 11th Floor, New York, NY 10016; (212) 252-8584

http://www.autismspeaks.org

Autism Society of America

7910 Woodmont Avenue, Suite 650, Bethesda, MD 20814;
   (301) 657-0881

http://www.autism-society.org/

Autistic Children's Activity Program

P.O. Box 4606, Portland, OR 97208; (503) 649-2066

Boy Scouts of America

1325 West Walnut Hill Lane, Irving, TX 75038; (972) 580-2000

Breckenridge Outdoor Education Center

P.O. Box 697, Breckenridge, CO 80424; (970) 453-6422

Camp Barnabas

901 Private Road 2060, Purdy, MO 65734; (417) 886-9800

www.campbarnabas.org

Camp Determination—Autism/Asperger Resource Center

4001 HC Miller Building—Kansas University Medical Ctr.
3901 Rainbow Blvd., Kansas City, KS 66160; (913) 588-5988

http://www.autismasperger.org

Camp Discovery

661 Ottowa Avenue, St. Paul, MN 55107

Camp for Children and Adults with Disabilities

9320 SW Barbur Blvd., Portland, OR 97219; (503) 452-7416

Camp Lee Mar

805 Redgate Road, Dresher, PA; (215) 658-1708 (winter)

450 Route 590, Lackawanna, PA; (570) 685-7188 (summer)

Challenger Sports Division

http://www.challenger-sports.org

Creative Living (Autism Society of NC)

1220 Nowell Road, Raleigh, NC 27607; (919) 854-6161

Gameclub

http://www.gameclubonline.com

Gateway Society Services for Persons with Autism

4807 Georgia Street, Delta, British Columbia, Canada V4K2T1

Girl Scouts of the United States of America

420 Fifth Avenue, New York, NY 10018; (800) 478-7248

http://www.girlscouts.org

Jay Nolan Community Services, Inc.

15501 San Fernando Mission Blvd., Suite 200, Mission Hills, CA 91345

http://www.jaynolan.org

National 4-H Council

7100 Connecticut Avenue, Chevy Chase, MD 20815

http://www.n4h.org

National Recreation and Park Association

22377 Belmont Ridge Road, Ashburn, VA 20148; (713) 858-0784

http://www.nrpa.org

National Sports Center for the Disabled

P.O. Box 1290, Winter Park, CO 80482; (970) 726-1540

National Therapeutic Recreation Society of the National Recreation and Park Association

22377 Belmont Ridge Road, Ashburn, VA 20148; (713) 858-0784
http://www.nrpa.org

North American Riding for the Handicapped Association

P.O. Box 33150, Denver, CO 80233; (303) 452-1212

Northern Suburban Special Recreation Program

3105 MacArthur Blvd., Northbrook, IL 60062; (847) 509-9400
http://www.nssra.org

Operation Access Project—Department of Recreation and Leisure

San Francisco State University, 1600 Holloway Avenue, San Francisco, CA 94132; (415) 338-0543

(The) Pilot House

P.O. Box 1553, Fairfield, CT 06825; (203) 610-3877
http://www.thepilothouse.org

Portland Bureau of Parks & Recreation—Disabled Citizens Recreation

1120 SW 5th Street, Portland, OR 97232; (503) 823-2525

Provincial Outreach Program for Autism and Related Disorders

4812 Georgia Street, Delta, British Columbia, Canada V4K2S9; (604) 946-3610

Specialized Recreation Program

2580 Hilyard Street, Eugene, OR 97405; (541) 682-5311
http://www.ci.eugene.or.us/rec

Special Olympics North America

1325 G. Street, NW, Suite 770, Washington, DC 20005; (202) 628-3630

Stepping Out Program at the Cove Center

866 Broadway, East Providence, RI 02914; (401) 438-4994

YMCA of the USA

101 North Wacker Drive, Chicago, IL 60606; (800) 872-9622
http://www.ymca.net

YWCA of the USA

1015 18th Street NW, Suite 1100, Washington, DC 20036;
  (202) 467-0801
http://www.ywca.org

INDEX